Diet Cheats Cookbook

D1121162

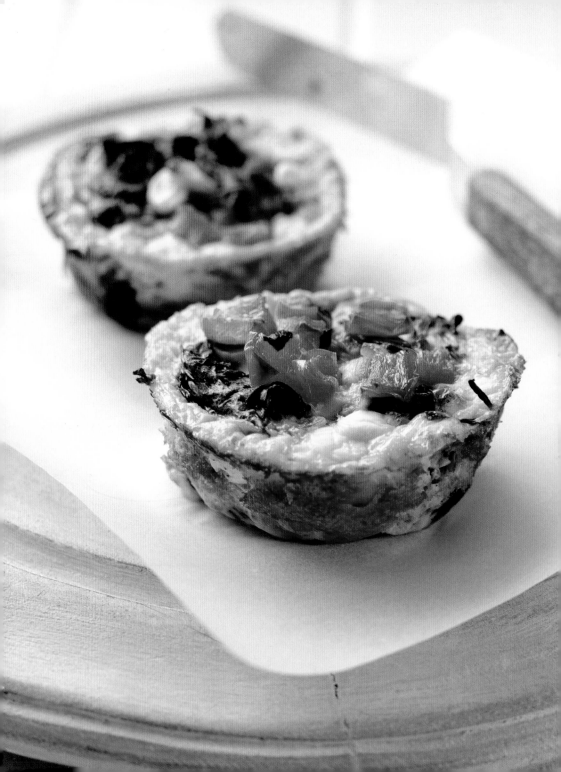

Diet Cheats Cookbook

Cook smart, satisfy cravings,
and lose weight forever!
100 guilt-free recipes

• • • • •

Heather Thomas

Vermilion
LONDON

1 3 5 7 9 10 8 6 4 2

Ebury Press, an imprint of Ebury Publishing,
20 Vauxhall Bridge Road,
London SW1V 2SA

Ebury Press is part of the Penguin Random House group of companies
whose addresses can be found at global.penguinrandomhouse.com

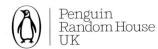

| Penguin
Random House
UK

Copyright © Ebury Press 2017
Photography by Joff Lee
Foor styling by Mari Williams
Design by Hugh Adams

First published by Ebury Press in 2018

www.eburypublishing.co.uk

A CIP catalogue record for this book is available from the British Library

ISBN 9781785037689

Printed and bound in China by Toppan Leefung

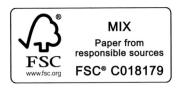

Contents

Introduction

The key to losing weight effectively is an eating plan that's simple to follow, enjoyable, sustainable, never leaves you feeling hungry and allows you to make your own choices about what you eat. In this book we take the hard work and stress out of dieting – there's no calorie counting and you decide what you want to eat. The quick and easy recipes enable you to eat a healthy diet with delicious food and good-sized portions that leave you feeling full for longer. You can navigate your way through the day without worrying about calories and quantities – there's no number crunching and it's easy to stay on course.

Traffic light colour-coded food lists

We have three colour-coded food lists (green, amber and red) to help you make the right choices.

- By choosing freely from the **green** list, you can stop worrying about what you're eating and proceed at your own pace, enjoying a wide range of healthy, nutritious foods. It's all about making smart choices.

- All the foods on the **amber** list can be eaten in moderation – not freely like the green foods. Amber foods tend to be higher in fat and calories but are still nutritious.

- Foods on the **red** list should be regarded with extreme caution and only eaten occasionally, if at all, as treats in very small quantities.

This healthy 'traffic lights' approach is easy to follow and it really works, and it's reflected in the recipes in this book. Just pick and mix your breakfasts/brunches, lunches, suppers, snacks and desserts – there's such a wide range that you're spoilt for choice. There are even special **cheat's** low-calorie slimming versions of many of your favourite dishes and take-out foods. You really can enjoy eating the foods you love but in a healthy, sustainable way.

Slimming success

If you want to be successful at losing unwanted pounds and maintaining a healthy weight long term, you need to learn new healthy eating habits and make them an intrinsic part of your lifestyle. It's not difficult – it's common sense.

1 Eat a healthy diet

You need to eat a varied diet with all the nutrients that are essential for good health, including lean protein (which includes vegetable protein from whole grains, pulses, beans, nuts); carbohydrates that are not over-refined and high in sugar (starchy vegetables, whole grains, brown rice, wholewheat pasta); vitamins and minerals; and, yes, even fat. Always opt for 'healthy' fats – monounsaturated olive oil, nuts, seeds and vegetable oils (in moderation on the amber list) rather than animal full-fat dairy products like cream and butter (red list). Most importantly, choose healthy foods you enjoy.

2 Eat 3-a-day

You should eat breakfast, lunch and dinner every day. If you go without food and miss meals, you'll crave it even more, your metabolism will slow, you'll have less energy and your health will suffer, so don't be tempted to skip breakfast or go without lunch.

3 Healthy snack attack

By eating regular healthy meals that fill you up you are less likely to feel hungry and be tempted to snack on foods that tend to be high in fat and sugar to give you a quick fix. But if you are still hungry, don't worry – you can choose a wide range of healthy options from the nutritious foods that can be eaten freely on the green list (see page 11) instead of filling up on unhealthy, high-calorie snacks and desserts. We also have delicious recipes for snacks (see page 107).

4 Eat less sugar and fat

Effective weight loss and maintenance are determined by the choices you make, so be smart and take control. Sugar is 'empty' calories and contributes nothing to your health and wellbeing. It's easy to reduce your intake: just choose sugarless or low-sugar foods and drinks and use natural plant-derived sweeteners, such as stevia. Learn which foods contain hidden sugar, including baked beans, ketchup, fruit yoghurts, fresh and canned soups, bread, breakfast cereals, smoothies and alcohol.

Fat (and that includes oils as well as the visible fat on meat and in dairy products, such as milk and cheese) has more calories than any other nutrient, so always make the smart choice and opt for healthy vegetable fats (nuts, avocados, seeds) and oils (e.g. olive and sunflower), oily fish and low-fat dairy foods. Remove the skin from chicken and all visible fat from meat.

Hidden sugar and fats

Sugar is often listed under other names, so check the label before buying and look for the following: corn syrup, dextrose, fructose, fruit sugar, glucose, lactose, maltose, molasses, sucrose, honey, agave syrup, maple syrup – they are all sugars. If you have a sweet tooth, enjoy the natural sweetness of fresh fruit and starchy vegetables, such as carrots, parsnips, swede and even peas, which are all **green** foods. Beware of packaged fruit juices as many contain added sugar and unwanted calories. It's better to eat an orange or squeeze one yourself.

Fats are sneaky and you may often eat them without even realising. Be aware of the hidden fats in mayonnaise, salad dressings and sauces as well as cookies, chocolate, desserts and snacks. Even 'healthy' yoghurts and smoothies can have a high fat content. Cook the low-fat way with low-cal spray oils and healthy cooking methods, including grilling (broiling), poaching and steaming.

5 Fill up with fibre

The dietary fibre in food makes you feel fuller for longer as well as playing an important role in promoting a healthy gut and digestive system. Eating high-fibre, low-GI (glycaemic index) foods (vegetables, fruit, beans, pulses, whole grains) that release energy slowly will reduce hunger pangs between meals, making you less likely to snack. GI ratings are given for all our recipes. Eat at least five portions of fruit and/or vegetables from the **green** list every day to boost your health and increase the fibre in your diet.

6 Treat yourself

Identify your trigger foods. We all have favourites that are hard to eat in moderation, especially when we need to spoil ourselves. You don't have to give them up – just enjoy them as an occasional treat to help you stay on track. When you reach a weight loss goal, a 'treat' will reward and motivate you.

Beware of 'empty' calories

You can drink alcohol as a treat but keep it for weekends and special occasions. Boost your weight loss, especially in the first few weeks, by staying alcohol-free. Alcohol is 'empty' calories – with virtually no nutrients and a high sugar content. If you drink just 5 small glasses of white wine a week, over the course of a month you will have consumed an extra 2,000 calories (kcals). That's 26,000 over the course of a year, which is an extra 3.6kg (8lb) of body fat (approximately, according to gender, height, build, age, etc.).

7 Don't obsess about your weight

Getting stressed about your weight and how slowly you're losing it is self-defeating. Successful weight loss takes time. If you crash diet and lose weight too fast, you're more likely to put it on again and there may be risks to your health. Eat the **green** foods and just relax and take it nice and easy. Weigh yourself once a week and record your weight loss in a diary. This will motivate you to eat healthily and keep on making the right choices. Weight can fluctuate on a daily basis due to hormonal changes and fluid retention in your body, so be smart and don't get on the scales every day.

8 Plan ahead

This can save you time and give you more control over the food you eat. By keeping a food diary or downloading an app onto your phone it's easier to track your eating habits, weight loss and which foods work for you. Plan your weekly meals in advance by writing a shopping list and doing one big shop or buying online instead of making several visits to the supermarket, where it's tempting to add less healthy foods to your trolley (cart). If you spend less time thinking about food, you have more to focus on other things in your life.

Social dieting

*You don't have to stop eating out – just make sensible choices and recognise the low-calorie healthy options on restaurant menus. As a general rule, salads, grilled (broiled) food, fish and chicken without creamy sauces are the best choices. Pasta is best eaten with a tomato-based sauce and you should avoid fried food. Plan ahead if you have a special dinner and eat really healthily in the preceding days. If you do over-indulge, don't worry. It's easy to get back on track if you eat mostly **green** foods (see page 11) in moderate portion sizes for a few days.*

9 Speed up your weight loss with exercise

Start exercising to burn fat and tone your body. Ideally, you need to exercise for at least 30 minutes four or five times a week. Choose an activity you enjoy and make it part of your way of life, so you're more likely to stick to it and it won't be just a passing fad. Walk or jog in the park, go for a cycle or a swim, join your local gym or dance class, whatever works for you. You can keep a record and measure the steps you take by downloading an app to your phone.

10 Stay slim

When you reach your goal, use our **green** and **amber** recipes to maintain your ideal weight. They're so simple to make and taste so good that you'll want to make them part of your everyday eating plan. By adopting a healthier diet in the long term you'll be more in control of what you eat and less likely to regain the pounds you've lost. Portion control is central to maintaining a healthy weight and it's so easy to do – you don't have to weigh everything obsessively. Just think of a plate and divide it into healthy food categories and portions – our user-friendly example shows you how.

HEALTHY EATING PLATE

Follow this basic principle when preparing meals to ensure you are getting the right nutrients and the correct portions to satisfy your cravings, and avoid the hidden calories that unclear portion sizes can contain.

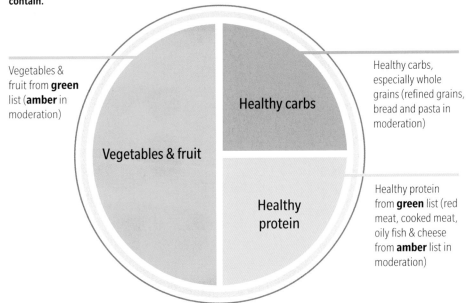

Vegetables & fruit from **green** list (**amber** in moderation)

Healthy carbs, especially whole grains (refined grains, bread and pasta in moderation)

Healthy carbs

Vegetables & fruit

Healthy protein

Healthy protein from **green** list (red meat, cooked meat, oily fish & cheese from **amber** list in moderation)

Smart cook

If you enjoy cooking from scratch and make it quick and easy, you'll make smart choices and be more in control of what you eat. You don't want to spend longer than you need to in the kitchen where the fridge and store cupboards offer tempting treats, so be savvy and follow the helpful guidelines set out below. You don't need specialist skills or know-how, just simple cooking methods and techniques. Instead of frying and roasting food in butter and oil, get used to cooking without the unwanted extra fat and calories – it's not difficult and it tastes just as good. All you need is low-cal spray oil – you can buy a one-calorie per spray brand in your local supermarket.

- **Baking and roasting:** When roasting or baking vegetables, chicken, meat and fish, just spray lightly with oil; 2–3 quick squirts will do the trick.
- **Grilling (broiling):** This is a healthy way to cook, especially when you're in a hurry. It uses hardly any oil and it's very fast. Use a conventional overhead grill, a ridged griddle pan, a barbecue or even buy a specially designed 'health grill' to channel fat away from the food into a drip tray.
- **Stir-frying:** One of the healthiest as well as the quickest way to cook. A whole meal can be cooked in a wok or deep frying pan in minimal oil. Use a branded one-calorie per spray oil or fill a misting oil sprayer with olive oil and keep it beside the hob.
- **Steaming:** This is the healthiest way to cook vegetables. It preserves their nutrients, colour, texture, crunchiness and flavour. Nothing is added, and the nutritional goodness is not leached into the cooking water, as happens when they are boiled.
- **Poaching:** To prevent chicken, salmon and white fish drying out and to keep them moist and tasty, you can poach them in water or stock in a pan on the hob or in a covered dish in the oven. No oil is needed.
- **Healthy flavourings:** Use herbs, spices, balsamic vinegar, lemon and lime, mustard and low-fat sauces to add depth and flavour without the calories.
- **Menu planning:** Plan your menus in advance and choose quick and easy dishes, so you don't spend more time than is necessary in the kitchen.
- **Stock up:** Always keep a selection of healthy foods and staples on the **green** foods list (see page 11) in your fridge, freezer and store cupboards, to avoid unnecessary shopping expeditions and temptation.
- **Refresh your fridge:** Keep a range of healthy, low-calorie foods you enjoy eating and like to cook. Throw away foods that are past their use-by date and any high-calorie ones on the red foods list (see page 13).
- **Top up the freezer:** Keep a selection of frozen healthy **green** foods, e.g. frozen berries, prawns, chicken breasts and sliced wholegrain bread for toasting (eat one slice at a time and use the defrost button on the toaster rather than having a whole loaf out on the counter). Label and freeze individual portions of healthy casseroles, soups, pasta sauces, etc., and reheat for quick meals.
- **Ready meals:** It's best to be in control of what you eat and prepare meals from scratch, but there will always be times when you can't cook, so keep a few healthy ready meals in the freezer. If you can quickly reheat a complete meal of less than 400–450 kcals per serving and eat it with salad or vegetables, you'll have a standby option. Always be sure to check the labels on ready meals carefully before buying, especially for fat content – ideally, they should be no higher than 5 per cent.

Eat yourself slim

The best way to eat yourself slim is to choose healthy, high-fibre, low-calorie foods you enjoy and which will fill you up, so you don't get hungry in between meals. There are lots of **green** foods you can eat for breakfast, lunch, dinner or snacks. They will:

- Stop you feeling hungry
- Help to fill you up
- Help you lose weight
- Make you feel more energised.

And the best bit is that you can eat them freely – as much of them as you like – without gaining weight. All our recipes feature these good-to-go **green** foods, and they are listed below.

The **green** foods don't include healthy carbs. You should still eat these every day but in moderation. These are included on the **amber** foods list (see page 12). As a general rule, the **amber** foods should never take up more than one-quarter of what's on your plate – the other three-quarters should be **green** foods (see diagram on page 9).

Lastly, there are **red** foods that are so high in sugar or fat that you should stop and think carefully before choosing them. Either avoid them altogether or eat only occasionally as treats. Use our helpful guide to identify them for quick and easy reference (see page 13).

....

Green foods – good to go!
Eat these foods freely – you don't need to weigh or measure them

Poultry: chicken and turkey (skin removed), grilled (broiled), poached or roasted with spray oil (not fried)

Fish and shellfish: all white fish, grilled (broiled), baked or steamed; tuna (fresh or canned in spring water); smoked salmon; trout; canned sardines in tomato sauce or brine (not oil); squid, grilled (broiled) not fried; mussels, clams, oysters, scallops, prawns (shrimp), white crabmeat, lobster

Eggs: all eggs (not fried)

Vegetarian protein foods: Quorn mince, fillets and chunks, tofu (bean curd)

Dairy and cheese: skimmed milk, low-fat soya milk, unsweetened almond milk; 0% fat probiotic drinks; 0% fat plain Greek yoghurt, very low-fat yoghurt (75 kcals max); low-fat cottage cheese, extra light soft cheese, Quark, virtually fat-free fromage frais

Pulses and beans: lentils (Puy, green, brown, red); green and yellow split peas; dried and canned beans, including black, black-eyed, borlotti, butterbeans (lima beans), cannellini, chickpeas, haricot, kidney beans

Vegetables: alfalfa, asparagus, artichokes, aubergine (eggplant), baby whole sweetcorn, bamboo shoots, bean sprouts, beetroot (beets), broccoli, Brussels sprouts, butternut squash, cabbage, carrots, cauliflower, celeriac, celery, chicory (Belgian endive), chillies, Chinese leaves (Chinese cabbage), courgettes (zucchini), cucumber, endive, fennel, fine green beans, garlic, gherkins, ginger, green beans, kale, leeks, lettuce, mange tout (snow peas), mushrooms, mustard & cress, okra, onions, pak choi (bok choy), parsnips, peas, (bell) peppers, pumpkin, radicchio, radishes, rocket (arugula), runner beans, seaweed, shallots, spinach, spring onions (scallions), sugar snap peas, swede (rutabaga), fresh tomato salsa, tomatoes (fresh and canned, not sun-dried), turnips, vine leaves, water chestnuts, watercress

Fresh fruit: apples, apricots (not dried), blackberries, blackcurrants, blueberries, cherries, clementines, cranberries (not dried), dates (fresh), gooseberries, grapefruit, kiwi, lemons, limes, lychees, mandarins, mango, melon, nectarines, oranges (not juice), papaya, passion fruit, peaches, pears, pineapple, plums, pomegranate, raspberries, rhubarb, satsumas, strawberries, tangerines, watermelon

Herbs and spices: all dried and fresh herbs and spices (whole or ground), curry powder (not curry paste)

Bakery: high-fibre crispbreads and crackers with less than 5% fat, rice cakes

Snacks and sweets: no-sugar jelly

Spreads: Marmite, Bovril, Vegemite, yeast extract, sugar-free jam and marmalade

Oils: low-calorie spray oil, olive oil sprays

Dressings and sauces: oil-free vinaigrette and salad dressings, extra light mayonnaise, soy sauce, teriyaki sauce, nam pla (Thai fish sauce), mint sauce (no added sugar), Tabasco sauce, oyster sauce, Worcestershire sauce, harissa paste

Condiments: artificial sweeteners, e.g. stevia, mustard, vinegars, low-fat stock cubes

Drinks: water, tea and coffee (plain or with skimmed milk), herbal and fruit tea, zero-calorie soft drinks

....

Amber foods – go slow!
Eat these foods in moderation unless instructed otherwise

Meat: extra lean beef, lamb, pork, veal (all visible fat removed), grilled (broiled) or roasted with spray oil; extra lean minced beef (less than 5% fat); liver, kidneys; low-fat sausages, low-fat beefburgers

Cooked meat: ham and gammon (all visible fat removed), Parma and serrano ham (cut wafer thin and visible fat removed), lean back bacon rashers (slices), all visible fat removed, turkey rashers

Poultry: duck (all skin removed)

Fish and shellfish: fresh salmon, herring, mackerel, sardines, grilled (broiled), baked or poached, no more than twice weekly; sushi

Dairy and cheese: semi-skimmed milk, low-fat yoghurt (over 75 kcals), half- or reduced-fat crème fraîche, low-fat ice cream; reduced-fat Cheddar, low-fat mozzarella and feta; light soft cheese, grated Parmesan on pasta (no more than 1 tsp max), low-fat spread

Breakfast cereals: unsweetened high-fibre cereals such as Weetabix, Shredded Wheat (not filled), oatmeal, porridge oats, unsweetened muesli, granola

Pasta and noodles: all plain varieties (dry, not fresh) boiled, in small quantities (no more than 90g/3oz cooked weight)

Rice: brown, basmati, Thai fragrant, Arborio and risotto rice, boiled or steamed, in small quantities (no more than 90g/3oz cooked weight)

Whole grains: bulgur wheat, quinoa, couscous, spelt, barley, pearl barley in small quantities (no more than 90g/3oz cooked weight)

Nuts: chestnuts, peanuts, cashews, pecans, walnuts, Brazil nuts, hazelnuts, pistachios, almonds (1 small handful max); pine nuts (1 tbsp max); coconut (15g/½oz max); reduced-fat coconut milk (50ml/2fl oz max)

Seeds: pumpkin, sesame, flaxseeds, sunflower, chia (1 tbsp max)

Vegetables: potatoes, sweet potatoes, yams, plantains, boiled, baked or dry-roasted; olives; sweetcorn (fresh or canned in natural spring water); sunblush and sun-dried tomatoes

Fresh fruit: 1 medium banana, grapes (15 max), ½ small avocado

Dried fruits: figs, dates, apricots, prunes, cranberries, raisins, sultanas, currants, mango, pineapple (30g/1oz max)

Prepared salads: coleslaw, potato salad, beetroot (beet) salad, Russian salad, couscous salad (small portions only)

Pastry: filo (phyllo), brushed with beaten egg or lightly sprayed with oil

Bakery: wholemeal and multi-grain bread (2 slices max), muffins, tortillas, wraps, pitta bread, oatcakes, plain crackers, sandwiches (no more than 350 kcals and 5% fat max)

Desserts, spreads and sweets: meringues, fruit salad in unsweetened natural juice, low-sugar jam, honey (1 heaped tsp max)

Dressings and sauces: Thai sweet chilli sauce, extra light and light mayonnaise, mango chutney, tomato ketchup, horseradish sauce, low-fat custard, green and red pesto (1 tsp only), curry paste

Oils and spreads: olive or sunflower oil (1 tsp max); reduced- or low-fat sunflower/olive oil spread (1 thin 7g/¼oz spread max)

Drinks: pure unsweetened fruit juices (drink in moderation as many are naturally high in sugar); fruit smoothies; low-sugar fruit squash, cordials and flavoured drinks; alcohol (light beer, wine, spirits), soda water, sparkling mineral water or low-calorie mixers; skinny low-fat cappuccino and latte

....

Red foods – stop and think!
Avoid the following or eat only occasionally
as treats in very small quantities

Meat: sausages (with more than 5% fat), spare ribs, belly pork

Cooked meats: salami, chorizo, peperoni, pâté

Fish: deep-fried battered fish, scampi and calamari

Dairy and cheese: full-fat milk, cream, soured cream, crème fraîche; full-fat ice cream; sweetened full-fat creamy yoghurts; full-fat and creamy cheeses, e.g. blue cheese, Brie, Camembert, cream cheese; full-fat Cheddar

Pasta and noodles: pasta in creamy sauces, fried noodles, gnocchi, filled pasta (tortelloni, ravioli, etc.)

Rice: fried rice and arancini (rice balls)

Oats: porridge with cream or full-fat milk and sugar

Breakfast cereals: sweetened brands, granola, cereal bars with a high sugar content and more than 5% fat

Nuts: peanut butter and nut spreads; nut brittle; satay sauce; creamed coconut, full-fat coconut milk

Vegetables: fried or battered vegetables, e.g. French fries and onion rings

Fruit: fruit canned in syrup or candied

Confectionery (candy) and spreads: chocolate bars, chocolate spreads, sweets (candy), candied popcorn; jam and marmalade (made with sugar)

Bakery: croissants, brioche, doughnuts, Danish pastries, cakes, scones, most muffins (check calorie content); pizza (especially deep pan)

Pastry: shortcrust, flaky, puff, hot water-crust, choux; pork pies; quiches

Snacks and sweets: potato crisps (chips), tortilla chips, biscuits and cookies; sugar, maple syrup, golden syrup, molasses, treacle; most desserts, especially cheesecake, pies, tarts

Dressings and sauces: creamy full-fat sauces, hollandaise, Béarnaise, tartare, full-fat mayonnaise, salad cream, oily and creamy salad dressings, e.g. blue cheese, thousand island, vinaigrette made with oil, guacamole, full-fat hummus, taramasalata

Oils and fats: olive, sunflower, rapeseed, coconut, vegetable, avocado, grapeseed, sesame and corn oils; butter, lard (shortening), dripping, margarine, ghee

Drinks: fortified wines, liqueurs, beer and cider, cocktails, sweetened soft drinks, e.g. cola; full-fat latte and cappuccino

Treats

In addition, you can have 2 **treats** per day max. They should be less than 200 kcals max (preferably 100 kcals) and can be **amber** or **red** foods. Try the following:

- A sugar-free jelly for when you're craving a dessert
- A small handful of dried fruit for a quick sweet snack
- A small handful of salted peanuts, mini pretzels or some salted popcorn when you fancy something salty
- A square of dark chocolate when you're really craving and missing chocolate bars
- A slimline G+T or glass of dry white wine when you're relaxing at the weekend or eating out on special occasions

Note: We have recipes for 100 kcals and 200 kcals treats you can make at the end of this book (see page 106).

You don't have to reward yourself with food when you achieve the goals you set yourself as you progress on your journey to your target weight. For instance, you could buy a new smaller pair of jeans, have a day out or a weekend break, book a special dinner, invest in a gym membership or join a dance class.

Healthy swaps and smart choices

To lose weight and stay that way permanently, you need to make healthy lifestyle and diet changes. This means recognising smart food choices and swapping unhealthy or high-calorie foods for healthier, lower-calorie ones that taste equally delicious. Nothing could be easier! Making healthy swaps will soon become second nature to you. These principles are exemplified best by our special **cheat's** recipes, which are featured in every section.

- Use spray oil for cooking food: one spray equates to one calorie. You can buy a low-cal spray or put some healthy olive oil in a non-aerosol refillable spray bottle and keep it handy beside the hob.
- Instead of French fries with chicken or a steak, make some baked butternut squash or swede (rutabaga) 'fries'.
- Serve pasta in a tomato sauce, not a creamy one.
- Boil or steam vegetables instead of frying them.
- Use reduced-fat or half-fat instead of regular full-fat cheeses.
- Use reduced-fat coconut milk in curries – you won't notice the difference.
- Substitute skimmed milk or unsweetened almond milk or soy milk for full-fat or semi-skimmed.
- Use 0% fat Greek yoghurt to make dips, desserts and sauces.
- Make sauces creamy by stirring in a spoonful of low-fat yoghurt, virtually fat-free fromage frais or half-fat crème fraîche at the end instead of cream.
- Instead of sugar, use fruit or artificial sweeteners; or balsamic vinegar in tomato sauce and salad dressings.
- Thicken sauces with cornflour (cornstarch) and water or skimmed milk instead of flour and butter.
- Bulk out soups and salads with healthy high-fibre beans and lentils rather than serving them with bread.
- Swap regular Indian tonic for slimline tonic as a mixer with gin or vodka (it's less than half the calories).
- Choose diet cola, lemonade and other soft drinks rather than the regular brands sweetened with sugar.
- Swap full-fat cappuccino and latte for low-fat skinny versions made with skimmed milk or unsweetened almond and soya milk.
- Instead of a sweet dessert, finish your meals with a piece of fresh fruit from the **green** food list or a low-fat (less than 100 kcals and 5% fat) yoghurt or 0% fat Greek yoghurt.

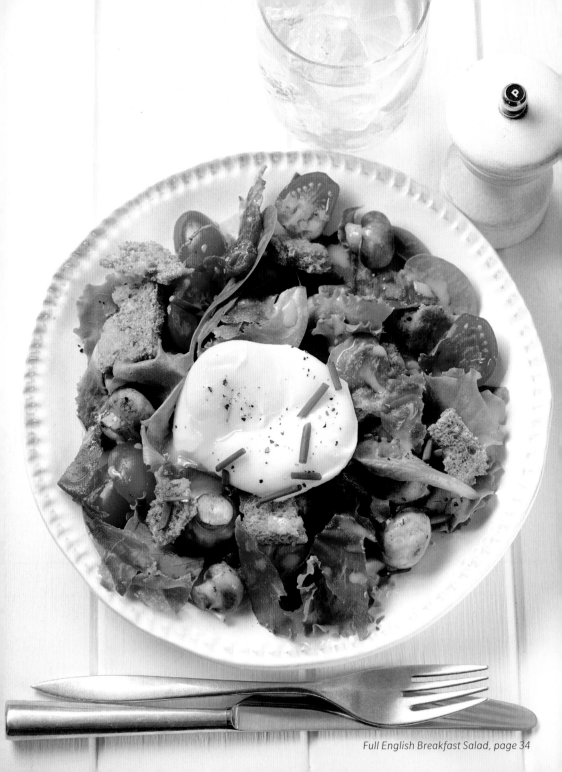

Full English Breakfast Salad, page 34

Start the day right

(breakfasts & brunches)

GREEN RECIPES (MAX 200 KCALS)	AMBER RECIPES (MAX 250 KCALS)
Fruity kale smoothie	Powerstart smoothies
Mango and carrot smoothie	Healthkick smoothie
Orange stewed rhubarb with cinnamon yoghurt	Herby French toast
Boiled eggs with veggie dippers	Fruity chia seed 'porridge'
Baked spinach and tomato eggs	Cheat's low-calorie granola
Piperade	Cheat's blueberry muffins
Huevos rancheros	Full English breakfast salad
Cheat's breakfast quiches	Egg, tomato and mushroom crumpet stacks
Smoked salmon and chives scrambled eggs	Cheat's breakfast burritos
Spinach and mushrooms with poached eggs	All-day breakfast omelette
Cheat's skinny English breakfast	Cheat's sweet potato 'toast' with smashed avocado with alternative toppings

KICKSTART SMOOTHIES

Smoothies are not only a great way to start the day but also provide some of the healthy fruit and vegetables you need to meet your 5-a-day target. These ones are made without bananas, which are not 'free' (green), but they are equally thick and creamy. For extra flavour, try adding a pinch of ground cinnamon or nutmeg or a few drops of vanilla extract.

Fruity kale smoothie

SERVES 2

Prep: 10 minutes

Per serving:

170 kcals

711 kJ

1.6g fat

Low GI

50g/2oz kale, washed and stalks removed

½ cucumber

2.5cm/1in fresh root ginger, peeled and chopped

a few sprigs of mint or parsley

1 apple, cored and sliced

2 slices fresh pineapple, peeled

125g/4oz (generous ¾ cup) frozen blueberries

4 tbsp 0% fat Greek yoghurt

150ml/¼ pint (generous ½ cup) unsweetened almond milk

1 Place the kale, cucumber, ginger and herbs in a blender. Add the apple, pineapple and blueberries and then blitz briefly until thick and smooth.

2 Add the yoghurt and pulse until well blended.

3 Pour into 2 glasses and drink immediately.

Mango *and* carrot smoothie

1 large mango

2 large carrots, peeled and chopped

300g/10oz galia melon, peeled, deseeded and chopped

1 tsp ground turmeric

2 large oranges, peeled and segmented

180ml/6fl oz (¾ cup) unsweetened soya milk

1 Peel the mango and remove the stone. Chop the flesh and place in a blender with the carrots, melon, turmeric and orange segments.

2 Blitz on high until thick and smooth, then add the soya milk and blitz again until well blended.

3 Pour into glasses and serve – with ice, if wished.

SERVES 2

Prep: 10 minutes

Per serving:

180 kcals

753 kJ

2.3g fat

Low GI

ORANGE STEWED RHUBARB *with* CINNAMON YOGHURT

There's no added sugar in this colourful dish – only the natural sweetness of the dates and orange juice. If you have a really sweet tooth you could drizzle each portion with a teaspoon of clear honey but it's not a 'free' (green) food and will add 18 kcals. Serve the rhubarb as a topping for 'porridge' (see page 31) or to have with granola (see page 32).

SERVES 2

Prep: 10 minutes

Cook: 8–10 minutes

Per serving:

190 kcals

795 kJ

0.3g fat

Medium GI

350g/12oz pink rhubarb, trimmed and cut into chunks

60g/2oz (¼ cup) fresh dates, stoned (pitted) and chopped

grated zest and juice of 1 large orange

1 tsp finely grated fresh root ginger

1 tbsp water

1 vanilla pod bean, split lengthways

350g/12oz (1½ cups) 0% fat Greek yoghurt

¼ tsp ground cinnamon

1 Put the rhubarb in a saucepan with the dates, orange zest and juice, ginger and water. Bring to the boil, then reduce the heat to a bare simmer and cook for about 5 minutes until the rhubarb is just tender but not mushy – it should hold its shape. Set aside to cool a little or leave to go cold and store overnight in a sealed container for tomorrow's breakfast.

2 With the sharp tip of a knife, scrape the vanilla seeds out of the pod into the yoghurt and stir well.

3 Divide the yoghurt between 2 bowls and spoon the warm or cold rhubarb over the top. Dust with cinnamon and serve.

BOILED EGGS *with* VEGGIE DIPPERS

Crisp blanched green vegetable dippers make a delicious and very healthy low-fat alternative to buttered toast. Choose plain crispbreads without seeds or cheese as they can pack a lot of extra calories. Check the labels carefully and make sure you use extra light soft cheese – it has one-third less fat and calories than light soft cheese.

SERVES 2

Prep: 10 minutes

Cook: 4 minutes

Per serving:

190 kcals

795 kJ

7.7g fat

Medium GI

100g/3½oz asparagus spears, trimmed

100g/3½oz tenderstem broccoli spears, trimmed

100g/3½oz fine green beans, topped and tailed

sea salt and freshly ground black pepper

2 medium free-range eggs

2 x 10g/⅓oz wholegrain or rye crispbreads

60g/2oz (½ cup) extra light soft cheese

1 Blanch the asparagus, broccoli and green beans in a pan of boiling water for 2–3 minutes until just tender but still firm. Remove gently with a slotted spoon, then drain on kitchen paper (paper towels) and season lightly with salt and pepper.

2 Meanwhile, boil the eggs in another pan of water for 4 minutes, to give you whites that are set but yolks that are still runny.

3 Cut the tops off the eggs and serve immediately with the vegetable dippers and the crispbreads spread with the soft cheese.

BAKED SPINACH
and TOMATO EGGS

This healthy brunch is really quick and easy to prepare and cook. You can spice it up by adding a pinch of dried chilli flakes or a dash of Tabasco. If you don't have any fresh spinach, use frozen instead – the calories will stay the same.

SERVES 2

Prep: 10 minutes

Cook: 15 minutes

Per serving:

200 kcals

837 kJ

7.4g fat

Low GI

500g/1lb 2oz spinach, washed and trimmed

a pinch of grated nutmeg

sea salt and freshly ground black pepper

low-cal spray oil

4 spring onions (scallions), chopped

200g/7oz small cherry or baby plum tomatoes, halved

2 medium free-range eggs

4 tbsp 0% fat Greek yoghurt

a small handful of dill, chopped

1 Preheat the oven to 190°C, 375°F, gas mark 5.

2 Put the damp spinach in a large saucepan over a medium heat. Cover with a lid and cook for 1–2 minutes, shaking the pan occasionally, until the spinach wilts and turns bright green. Alternatively, pour some boiling water over the spinach in a colander or wilt in the microwave.

3 Drain well in a colander, pressing down with a saucer to squeeze out any excess water. Pat dry with kitchen paper (paper towels) and chop coarsely. Season with nutmeg, salt and pepper.

4 Lightly spray a flameproof casserole dish with oil and set over a low to medium heat. Add the spring onions and tomatoes and cook for 2–3 minutes, then stir in the spinach and cook for 1 minute. Remove from the heat and make 2 hollows in the spinach. Break an egg into each one.

5 Bake in the preheated oven for about 10 minutes until the egg whites are set but the yolks are still runny.

6 Remove from the oven and spoon the yoghurt over the top. Sprinkle with dill and a grinding of black pepper and serve immediately.

PIPERADE

This traditional dish comes from the Basque region in southwest France and is a colourful, more substantial version of scrambled eggs. Piperade is very versatile and you can use canned tomatoes instead of fresh, and chopped parsley instead of basil. The French use only green (bell) peppers but you can substitute red or yellow ones if preferred.

SERVES 2

Prep: 10 minutes

Cook: 20–25 mins

Per serving:

200 kcals

837 kJ

8.8g fat

Low GI

low-cal spray oil

1 onion, thinly sliced

2 garlic cloves, crushed

2 green (bell) peppers, deseeded and thinly sliced

½ tsp hot or smoked paprika

3 ripe tomatoes, skinned and chopped

sea salt and freshly ground black pepper

3 medium free-range eggs

a few basil leaves, chopped

1 Lightly spray a large non-stick frying pan (skillet) with oil and set over a low heat. Add the onion, garlic and peppers and cook gently for 8–10 minutes until really tender.

2 Stir in the paprika and tomatoes and increase the heat to medium. Cook for about 10 minutes until the sauce reduces and the liquid evaporates. Season to taste with salt and pepper. Remove about three-quarters of the mixture from the pan and keep warm.

3 Beat the eggs in a bowl with a little salt and pepper. Pour into the frying pan and stir with a wooden spoon over a low heat until they start to set and scramble. Take care not to overcook them – they should be creamy. Remove the pan from the heat.

4 Gently stir the scrambled eggs and basil into the reserved warm tomato mixture, and divide between 2 serving plates. Eat immediately.

HUEVOS RANCHEROS

Eat these Mexican-style baked eggs for a weekend brunch or even for supper. You can use orange or yellow (bell) peppers instead of red and the calories will stay the same. If you like hot food, you can make this dish more fiery, by adding a diced red chilli with the onion.

SERVES 2

Prep: 10 minutes

Cook: 25–30 mins

Per serving:

190 kcals

795 kJ

6.3g fat

Low GI

low-cal spray oil

1 red onion, finely chopped

1 garlic clove, crushed

2 red (bell) peppers, deseeded and diced

a pinch of dried chilli flakes

1 x 400g/14oz can (scant 2 cups) chopped tomatoes

150ml/¼ pint (generous ½ cup) vegetable stock

sea salt and freshly ground black pepper

2 medium free-range eggs

a few sprigs of coriander (cilantro), chopped

1 Preheat the oven to 180°C, 350°F, gas mark 4.

2 Lightly spray a frying pan (skillet) with oil and set over a low to medium heat. Cook the onion, garlic and red peppers, stirring occasionally, for 8–10 minutes until tender.

3 Reduce the heat and add the chilli flakes, tomatoes and stock. Cook gently for 6–8 minutes until the mixture reduces and thickens. Season to taste with salt and pepper.

4 Divide between 2 small ovenproof dishes and make a small indentation in the centre of each one with the back of a spoon. Crack an egg into the hollow and bake in the preheated oven for about 10 minutes until the eggs are cooked and set.

5 Serve immediately, sprinkled with coriander.

CHEAT'S BREAKFAST QUICHES

These healthy no-pastry 'quiches' can be eaten hot or cold for breakfast, as snacks or even a packed lunch. A single one is only 99 kcals and packed with nutritional goodness. You can substitute cooked diced mushrooms, leeks or courgette (zucchini) for the (bell) pepper and tomatoes, or parsley for the chives.

SERVES 2

Prep: 15 minutes

Cook: 30 minutes

Per serving (2 quiches):

198 kcals

828 kJ

7.1g fat

Low GI

low-cal spray oil

1 small red onion, finely chopped

1 large red or yellow (bell) pepper, deseeded and diced

2 medium tomatoes, chopped

200g/7oz baby spinach leaves

2 medium free-range eggs

4 tbsp skimmed milk

1 small bunch of chives, snipped

100g/3½oz (scant ½ cup) low-fat cottage cheese

sea salt and freshly ground black pepper

1 Preheat the oven to 190°C, 375°F, gas mark 5.

2 Lightly spray a non-stick frying pan (skillet) with oil and set over a medium heat. Add the red onion and pepper and cook for 6–8 minutes until softened. Add the tomatoes and spinach and cook for 2 minutes until the spinach wilts and turns bright green. Remove from the heat and set aside.

3 Lightly spray 4 hollows of a non-stick muffin tin (pan) with oil and divide the vegetable mixture between them.

4 In a bowl, beat together the eggs and milk. Stir in the chives and cottage cheese, and season to taste.

5 Pour the egg mixture over the vegetables and bake in the preheated oven for about 20 minutes until the quiches have risen and are golden brown on top and firm to the touch. If you aren't eating them warm, set aside to cool and then store in a container in the fridge to enjoy the following day.

SMOKED SALMON *and* CHIVES SCRAMBLED EGGS

You don't need to use lots of butter to make good scrambled eggs – just some spray oil and a good-quality non-stick saucepan. If you want to serve them with toast, remember that an unbuttered average 40g/1½oz slice of wholemeal bread will add around 90 kcals per serving. And even a thinly spread scraping of butter (7g/¼oz) will add another 51 kcals and a whopping 5.7g fat! Better to serve this with some plain grilled tomatoes and mushrooms from the 'green' list.

SERVES 2

Prep: 5 minutes

Cook: 2–3 minutes

Per serving:

210 kcals

879 kJ

14g fat

Low GI

4 medium free-range eggs

1 small bunch of chives, snipped

sea salt and freshly ground black pepper

low-cal spray oil

50g/2oz smoked salmon, diced

1 tbsp half-fat crème fraîche

1 Break the eggs into a bowl. Add the chives and a little salt and pepper, just enough to season them. Beat with a fork or a balloon whisk until the yolks and whites are combined.

2 Lightly spray a small non-stick saucepan with oil and set over a medium heat. Add the eggs to the hot pan, then reduce the heat and stir gently for 2–3 minutes, drawing in the mixture from the sides of the pan, until they start to scramble and set. They should be creamy and slightly runny.

3 Quickly stir in the smoked salmon and crème fraîche. Don't overcook the eggs – they will continue cooking even after you've taken them off the heat. Transfer them to 2 warm serving plates and serve immediately.

SPINACH *and* MUSHROOMS *with* POACHED EGGS

SERVES 2

Prep: 10 minutes

Cook: 25 minutes

Per serving:

150 kcals

628 kJ

7.4g fat

Low GI

Cooking the mushrooms in vegetable stock instead of oil makes them really flavoursome, tender and almost syrupy. You could add finely shredded kale instead of spinach and cook for an extra 2–3 minutes. Serve with 2 low-fat rice cakes and you will have a really delicious and healthy 200-calorie breakfast or brunch.

250g/9oz mushrooms, thinly sliced

240ml/8fl oz (1 cup) vegetable stock

200g/7oz baby spinach leaves

sea salt and freshly ground black pepper

2 x 85g/3oz sprigs of cherry tomatoes on the vine

1 tsp white wine vinegar

2 medium free-range eggs

balsamic vinegar for drizzling

a few chives, snipped

1 Put the mushrooms and stock in a saucepan, cover with a lid and bring to the boil. Boil for 5 minutes, then uncover the pan and simmer gently for about 20 minutes until the liquid has evaporated and the mushrooms are really tender and golden brown.

2 Stir in the spinach and cook gently over a low heat for 1–2 minutes or until the leaves wilt and turn bright green. Season to taste with salt and pepper.

3 Preheat the grill (broiler) until hot, then grill the cherry tomato sprigs for 3–4 minutes until they start to soften and the skins change colour.

4 Meanwhile, to poach the eggs, bring a small saucepan of water to the boil, then reduce the heat to a bare simmer, add the vinegar and gently break the eggs into the hot water. Cover the pan and leave to cook over the lowest possible heat for about 3–4 minutes until the whites are set but the yolks are still runny. Remove with a slotted spoon and drain on kitchen paper (paper towels).

5 Divide the spinach and mushrooms between 2 warm serving plates. Drizzle with balsamic vinegar and top with a warm poached egg. Sprinkle with chives and serve.

CHEAT'S SKINNY ENGLISH BREAKFAST

SERVES 2

Prep: 5 minutes

Cook: 8 minutes

Per serving:

200 kcals

837 kJ

8.9g fat

Low GI

This is our delicious low-calorie cheat's version of the full English breakfast. If wished, you can poach the eggs instead of cooking them in the pan. Vegetarians can substitute Quorn bacon-style slices for the turkey rashers (turkey bacon strips). Use chestnut mushrooms if you can get them – they have a better flavour than the white closed cup or button varieties. Serve each portion with a 25g/1oz slice of wholemeal toast and you'll add 58 kcals.

2 ripe medium tomatoes, halved

4 turkey rashers (turkey bacon strips)

sea salt and freshly ground black pepper

low-cal spray oil

175g/6oz mushrooms, e.g. chestnut or closed cap

2 large free-range eggs

2 tsp tomato ketchup

1 Preheat the grill (broiler) and place the tomato halves, cut side up, and the turkey rashers on a foil-lined grill pan. Grind a little black pepper over the tomatoes.

2 Cook under the hot grill for about 5 minutes, turning the turkey rashers over halfway through. Keep warm.

3 Meanwhile, lightly spray a non-stick frying pan (skillet) with oil and set over a medium heat. Add the mushrooms and cook on both sides for 4–5 minutes until tender and golden brown. Remove and keep warm.

4 Gently break the eggs into the hot pan and cook until the whites are set and the yolks are still runny. To cook the top, you can pop the pan under the hot grill for 1–2 minutes.

5 Take 2 warm serving plates and divide the tomatoes, mushrooms, eggs and turkey rashers between them. Season, if wished, with salt and pepper and serve with the tomato ketchup.

POWERSTART SMOOTHIES

SERVES 2

Prep: 5 minutes

A thick smoothie is surprisingly filling and makes a big contribution towards your 5-a-day target. If wished, you can add a handful of chopped spinach or kale and a knob of fresh root ginger. The calories will only increase by approximately 10 per serving. If you're someone who's always in a rush in the morning and doesn't have time for breakfast, this is the perfect way to start your day.

Per serving:

250 kcals

1046 kJ

1.7g fat

Low GI

1 x 225g/8oz ripe mango

100g/3½oz strawberries

1 small banana

4 tbsp 0% fat Greek yoghurt

2 tbsp oat bran

1 tbsp ground flaxseeds

1 tsp clear honey

420ml/14fl oz (1¾ cups) skimmed milk or unsweetened soya milk

1 Peel the mango and cut the flesh from around the stone into chunks.

2 Place the mango, strawberries, banana, yoghurt, oat bran, seeds and honey in a blender. Add the milk.

3 Holding the lid of the blender firmly in place, blitz until everything is well combined and smooth. If the smoothie is too thick for your taste, add a little water to get the desired consistency.

4 Pour into 2 glasses and drink immediately. Alternatively, transfer to a jug and chill in the fridge for 1 hour – no longer or the banana will discolour.

> **TIP:** If you substitute unsweetened almond milk for soy or skimmed you will reduce the kcals per serving to 215.

HEALTH KICK SMOOTHIE

SERVES 1

Prep: 5 minutes

Per serving:

250 kcals

1046 kJ

2.5g fat

Low GI

Here's a really healthy fruit and vegetable smoothie to kick start your day. It's so simple to make – just put everything in a blender or food chopper and pulse until thick and smooth. We've added turmeric because it contains curcumin, which has anti-inflammatory and antioxidant properties. It also adds a lovely golden tinge to the smoothie. Don't be tempted to use more than the recommended amount (see below) or the flavour will dominate the natural sweetness of the orange juice, kiwi, strawberries and banana.

1 small banana, thickly sliced

60g/2oz whole strawberries, hulled

1 kiwi fruit, peeled and cut into chunks

50g/2oz small broccoli florets (raw), roughly chopped

125g/4oz (generous ½ cup) 0% fat Greek yoghurt

1 tsp pumpkin and/or sunflower seeds

½ tsp ground turmeric

60ml/2fl oz/¼ cup unsweetened orange juice

1 Put the banana, strawberries, kiwi fruit and broccoli in a blender or food chopper.

2 Add the yoghurt, seeds, turmeric and orange juice. Cover with the lid and blitz briefly until thick and smooth. If it's too thick for your liking, thin with a little water or skimmed milk.

3 Pour the smoothie into a large glass and enjoy!

Alternative flavourings:

You can use the following flavourings and the calories will stay roughly the same:

- Instead of using turmeric, add ¼ tsp ground cinnamon or a good grating of fresh nutmeg, or even a small piece of peeled fresh root ginger.

- Add a few drops of vanilla essence to taste.

- Use raw kale, spinach or spring greens instead of broccoli.

- Substitute fresh raspberries for the strawberries.

HERBY FRENCH TOAST

French toast is usually sweet, dusted with sugar and served with fruit and syrup, but our savoury version is healthier and even more delicious. If you love maple syrup, you can substitute it for the honey for no extra calories.

....

SERVES 2

Prep: 5 minutes

Soak: 2–3 minutes

Cook: 4–6 minutes

Per serving:

220 kcals

920 kJ

6.9g fat

Medium GI

2 medium free-range eggs

45ml/3 tbsp skimmed milk

a few sprigs each of parsley and chives, finely chopped

2 spring onions (scallions), very finely sliced

sea salt and freshly ground black pepper

2 x medium (44g/1½oz) slices seeded wholemeal bread

low-cal spray oil

2 x 85g/3oz bunches of cherry tomatoes on the vine

2 tsp clear honey

1 Beat the eggs and milk together in a shallow bowl. Add the herbs and spring onions. Season with a little salt and pepper.

2 Place the slices of bread in the eggy mixture and leave for 2–3 minutes to soak , turning the bread halfway through to cover both sides. It should absorb all the beaten egg.

3 Lightly spray a large non-stick frying pan (skillet) with oil and set over a low to medium heat. When the pan is really hot, carefully add the soaked bread slices and cook for 2–3 minutes until crisp and golden brown underneath. Turn them over and cook the other side.

4 Meanwhile, grill (broil) the tomatoes under a preheated hot grill (broiler) or cook on a griddle pan until slightly softened and charred.

5 Serve the hot French toast, drizzled with the honey, with the tomatoes on the side.

FRUITY CHIA SEED 'PORRIDGE'

Prepare this healthy breakfast the evening before and chill overnight in the fridge. By morning the chia seeds will swell to create a delicious 'porridge'. Chia is an excellent source of protein and fibre. It has a high fat content but it is omega-3 rich 'healthy' vegetable oil. You can use unsweetened soya milk instead of almond for an additional 15 kcals per serving. Or try strawberries, pomegranate seeds or blueberries instead of raspberries – the calories will stay the same. If you have a sweet tooth, a teaspoon of honey drizzled over each bowl will add 21 kcals per serving.

SERVES 2

Prep: 10 minutes

Chill: overnight

Per serving:

250 kcals

1046 kJ

12.2g fat

Low GI

---

1 large banana, mashed

4 tbsp chia seeds

300ml/½ pint (1¼ cups) unsweetened almond milk

2–3 drops of vanilla extract

a pinch of ground cinnamon

For the topping:

2 tsp pumpkin seeds

1 tbsp coconut flakes

100g/3½oz (scant 1 cup) raspberries

1 Put the mashed banana and chia seeds in a bowl and whisk in the milk until everything is well combined and there are no lumps of banana.

2 Set aside for 2–3 minutes, then whisk in the vanilla extract and cinnamon. The porridge should be starting to thicken already. Cover the bowl and leave to chill overnight in the fridge.

3 The following morning, the mixture should have thickened to a tapioca-like porridge. Divide it between 2 bowls, sprinkle with the pumpkins seeds and coconut flakes and top with the fresh raspberries.

CHEAT'S LOW-CALORIE GRANOLA

Most commercial brands of granola are loaded with fat and sugar and very high in calories, so it's better to make your own. This healthy recipe makes enough granola for 6 portions if served with skimmed milk or unsweetened soya or almond milk. Alternatively, you can sprinkle a little over some 0% fat Greek yoghurt and fresh fruit.

SERVES 6

Prep: 5 minutes

Cook: 20–25 minutes

Per serving:

190 kcals

795 kJ

10.6g fat

Low GI

1 tbsp coconut oil

1 tbsp maple syrup

100g/4oz (1¼ cups) rolled oats

30g/1oz (¼ cup) roughly chopped walnuts

2 tbsp sunflower seeds

2 tbsp pumpkin seeds

40g/1½oz (generous ¼ cup) raisins or dried cranberries

¼ tsp ground cinnamon

a few drops of vanilla extract

1 Preheat the oven to 170°C, 325°F, gas mark 3.

2 Heat the coconut oil and maple syrup in a pan set over a low heat until the coconut oil melts. Stir in the oats, walnuts, seeds, dried fruit, cinnamon and vanilla, making sure everything is well coated. Remove from the heat.

3 Pour the mixture in a thin layer over a large baking tray (cookie sheet), spreading it out evenly. Bake in the preheated oven for 15–20 minutes, stirring once or twice, until golden brown and crisp.

4 Set aside to cool and then transfer to an airtight container. Store in a cool, dry place for up to a month.

CHEAT'S BLUEBERRY MUFFINS

You can eat more of these high-fibre, moist muffins because they are made without fat and have less than half the calories of most shop-bought ones. Try adding different flavourings – orange zest or a few drops of vanilla extract – or serve them with a heaped spoonful of 0% fat Greek yoghurt for an extra 12 kcals. Ring the changes and substitute raspberries for the blueberries (the calories will stay the same).

MAKES 8 MUFFINS

Prep: 15 minutes

Soak: 10 minutes

Cook: 20 minutes

Per muffin:

100 kcals

1.5g fat

Medium GI

100ml/3½fl oz (scant ½ cup) skimmed milk

60g/2oz (scant ½ cup) wheat bran

60g/2oz (generous ¼ cup) soft brown sugar

1 large free-range egg

100g/3½oz (1 cup) plain (all-purpose) flour

½ tsp baking powder

½ tsp bicarbonate of soda (baking soda)

a pinch of ground cinnamon

a pinch of ground nutmeg

grated zest of 1 lemon

125g/4oz (1¼ cups) fresh blueberries

1 Preheat the oven to 190°C, 375°F, gas mark 5. Place 8 paper cases (muffin cases) in a muffin tin (pan).

2 Put the milk and wheat bran in a bowl and stir well. Set aside for 10 minutes to soak.

3 In another bowl, beat the sugar and egg together until creamy and well combined, then beat in the soaked milk and bran mixture. Sift in the flour, baking powder and bicarbonate of soda. Add the ground spices and lemon zest. Fold in gently with a metal spoon in a figure-of-eight motion. Stir in the blueberries, distributing them evenly throughout the mixture (batter).

4 Spoon the mixture into the paper cases and bake in the preheated oven for about 20 minutes or until the muffins have risen and are golden brown and firm to the touch.

5 Cool on a wire rack before eating. Or wrap in foil or a plastic bag and keep for 1–2 days at room temperature or 2–3 days in the fridge.

FULL ENGLISH BREAKFAST SALAD

This salad is an unusual and healthy twist on the traditional eggs and bacon breakfast. You can serve it as a light lunch or supper, too.

SERVES 2

Prep: 15 minutes

Cook: 10–12 minutes

Per serving:

250 kcals

1046 kJ

9g fat

Medium GI

4 x 15g/½oz slices Parma ham (prosciutto), all visible fat removed

spray olive oil

200g/7oz button mushrooms

100g/3½oz mixed salad leaves, e.g. rocket (arugula), frisée, chicory (Belgian endive)

8 cherry or baby plum tomatoes, halved or quartered

balsamic vinegar for drizzling (optional)

1 tsp white wine vinegar

2 medium free-range eggs

2 x 25g/1oz slices wholemeal bread

sea salt and freshly ground black pepper

snipped chives for sprinkling

For the mustardy dressing:

1 tbsp Dijon mustard

1 tbsp apple cider vinegar

2 tbsp water

1 level tsp clear honey or maple syrup

1 Heat a non-stick frying pan (skillet) over a low to medium heat and dry-fry the Parma ham for 2–3 minutes until crisp and golden brown. Drain on kitchen paper (paper towels) to absorb any fat.

2 Spray the pan lightly with oil and add the mushrooms. Cook for about 5 minutes until tender and golden brown all over.

3 Make the dressing: mix all the ingredients together in a bowl or shake in a screwtop jar until well blended. Gently toss the salad leaves, tomatoes and warm mushrooms in the dressing and divide between 2 serving plates. Drizzle with the balsamic vinegar, if you like.

4 Bring a small saucepan of water to the boil, then reduce the heat to a bare simmer, add the white wine vinegar and gently break the eggs into the hot water. Cover the pan and leave to cook over the lowest possible heat for about 3–4 minutes until the whites are set but the yolks are still runny. Remove with a slotted spoon and drain on kitchen paper.

5 Meanwhile, toast the bread and spray lightly with olive oil. Break into rough pieces.

6 Crumble the Parma ham over the salad and scatter with the pieces of toast. Top with a poached egg and season lightly with salt and pepper. Sprinkle with the chives and serve.

EGG, TOMATO *and* MUSHROOM CRUMPET STACKS

Even though crumpets are full of holes, they are quite filling and make a great base for a cooked breakfast. If you don't have them, you can substitute a split and toasted English muffin instead – the calories of half a muffin are approximately the same as those in a single crumpet.

SERVES 2

Prep: 5 minutes

Cook: 8–12 minutes

Per serving:

185 kcals

774 kJ

6g fat

Medium GI

---

low-cal spray oil

2 x 50g/2oz large flat mushrooms

1 large beefsteak tomato

1 tsp white wine vinegar

2 medium free-range eggs

2 x 40g/1½oz crumpets

2 tsp tomato ketchup

sea salt and freshly ground black pepper

chopped parsley for sprinkling

1 Lightly spray a large non-stick frying pan (skillet) with oil and set over a low to medium heat. Add the mushrooms to the hot pan and cook for about 5–8 minutes, turning them halfway through, until tender and golden brown. Remove and keep warm.

2 Cut the tomato in half horizontally and add to the pan. Cook for 3–4 minutes, turning once, until tender and starting to brown. Alternatively, you can cook the mushrooms and tomatoes under a hot overhead grill (broiler).

3 Meanwhile, bring a small saucepan of water to the boil, then reduce the heat to a bare simmer, add the vinegar and gently break the eggs into the hot water. Cover the pan and leave to cook over the lowest possible heat for about 3–4 minutes until the whites are set but the yolks are still runny. Remove with a slotted spoon and drain on kitchen paper (paper towels).

4 While the eggs are poaching, lightly toast the crumpets.

5 Assemble the stacks: spread the tomato ketchup over each toasted crumpet and place a tomato half on top. Add the mushrooms next (hollow side up) and fill each one with a poached egg. Grind over some salt and pepper and sprinkle with parsley. Serve immediately.

CHEAT'S BREAKFAST BURRITOS

Most burritos are very high in calories as they are served with lashings of sour cream and guacamole, but the good news is that you can make a healthy, slimming version for breakfast or brunch. To make these more filling, you can add some cherry tomatoes or mushrooms cooked in spray oil – the extra calories will be negligible.

SERVES 2

Prep: 10 minutes

Cook: 6–10 minutes

Per serving:

240 kcals

1004 kJ

9.4g fat

Medium GI

2 medium free-range eggs

a few sprigs of coriander (cilantro) or chives, chopped

sea salt and freshly ground black pepper

low-cal spray oil

4 spring onions (scallions), sliced

1 small red chilli, deseeded and diced

2 x 35g/1oz flour tortillas

4 tbsp low-fat salsa

2 tbsp grated low-fat Cheddar cheese

1 Whisk the eggs in a bowl with the chopped herbs and some salt and pepper.

2 Lightly spray a small non-stick frying pan (skillet) with oil and set over a low to medium heat. Add the spring onions and chilli and cook for 3–4 minutes until softened.

3 Reduce the heat to very low and pour the beaten eggs into the pan. Stir gently until they start to scramble and set. Remove from the heat immediately.

4 Meanwhile, warm the tortillas according to the instructions on the packet. You can do this in a low oven or on a hot griddle pan.

5 Spread the salsa over the warm tortillas and top with the scrambled egg mixture. Sprinkle with grated cheese and fold over or roll up. Eat immediately.

ALL-DAY BREAKFAST OMELETTE

The wonderful thing about this breakfast is that you can enjoy it at any time of the day. It's so easy to make and is a great way to use up leftover cooked potatoes from the night before. Vegetarians can substitute Quorn bacon-style rashers or slices for the bacon or sprinkle the omelette with 2 heaped tablespoons of grated reduced-fat Cheddar cheese before browning under the grill (broiler). The calories will stay the same.

SERVES 2

Prep: 5 minutes

Cook: 15–20 minutes

Per serving:

250 kcals

1046 kJ

12g fat

Medium GI

low-cal spray oil

100g/3½oz cooked new potatoes, diced

150g/5oz small mushrooms, quartered

50g/2oz thin-cut lean back bacon rashers (slices), all visible fat removed

8 cherry tomatoes, halved

4 medium free-range eggs

2 tbsp water

sea salt and freshly ground black pepper

1 small bunch of chives, snipped

1 Lightly spray a large non-stick frying pan (skillet) with oil and set over a medium heat. When the pan is hot, add the potatoes, mushrooms and bacon and cook for 5 minutes, turning occasionally, until the vegetables are tender and the bacon is golden brown and crisp. Add the tomatoes and cook for 2–3 minutes.

2 Beat the eggs and water together in a bowl. Season lightly with salt and pepper and beat in the chives.

3 Pour the beaten egg into the pan, swirling it around the vegetables and bacon. Reduce the heat and cook very gently for about 5 minutes until the omelette is set and golden brown underneath.

4 Meanwhile, preheat an overhead grill (broiler). When it's really hot, pop the omelette underneath for 2–3 minutes until the top is set and appetisingly browned.

5 Cut the omelette into wedges and divide between 2 serving plates. Eat immediately.

CHEAT'S SWEET POTATO 'TOAST' *with* SMASHED AVOCADO

Sweet potato 'toast' is a great way to start the day – it's low-calorie, healthy and nutritious. And it's so easy to make … just slice the sweet potatoes and pop them into a toaster. We've suggested three delicious toppings but you can have fun experimenting: try tzatziki (17 kcals per tbsp), hummus (25 kcals per tbsp), a mashed small banana (90 kcals) or a medium egg fried with a squirt of spray oil (76 kcals). Sprinkle with chopped herbs of your choice.

SERVES 2

Prep: 10 minutes

Cook: 3–5 minutes

Per serving:

190 kcals

795 kJ

9g fat

Low GI

2 tsp pine nuts

1 x 100g/3½oz (small) avocado

a squeeze of lemon or lime juice

a pinch of crushed chilli flakes (optional)

sea salt and freshly ground black pepper

1 x 200g/7oz (medium) sweet potato

8 baby plum tomatoes, halved

snipped chives for sprinkling

1 Heat a small frying pan (skillet) over a medium to high heat. When it's really hot, add the pine nuts and toss gently for 1–2 minutes until toasted and golden brown all over, watching them carefully to ensure that they don't catch and burn. Remove from the pan immediately.

2 Cut the avocado in half and remove the stone. Scoop out the flesh and mash coarsely with the lemon or lime juice and chilli flakes (if using). Season with salt and pepper.

3 Wash the sweet potato and pat dry with kitchen paper (paper towels). Cut lengthways into thin slices that will fit into your toaster – they should be no more than 5mm/¼in thick or they may not cook through. If you have a microwave, you could pop the slices in for 20–30 seconds before toasting, to be on the safe side.

4 Cook in the toaster until crisp and golden brown on the outside and soft on the inside. The time taken will depend on the thickness of the sweet potato and the setting on your toaster. You may have to toast it twice on medium to high to achieve the desired colour and degree of tenderness.

5 Spread the mashed avocado over the toasted sweet potato slices and top with the plum tomatoes. Sprinkle with the toasted pine nuts and chives and eat immediately.

Alternative toppings

SOFT CHEESE AND BLUEBERRIES

Spread the toast with 40g/1½oz (scant ¼ cup) extra light soft cheese and top with 80g/3oz fresh blueberries. Drizzle with balsamic vinegar.

Per serving: 130 kcals (544 kJ), 1.6g fat

Note: Drizzle each serving with 1 tsp maple syrup, adding 17 kcals

SMOKED SALMON AND SOFT CHEESE

Dice 100g/3½oz thinly sliced smoked salmon and mix with 40g/1½oz extra light soft cheese. Spread over the sweet potato toast, sprinkle with chopped dill and add a squeeze of lemon juice and a grinding of black pepper.

Per serving: 195 kcals (816 kJ) 6.5g fat

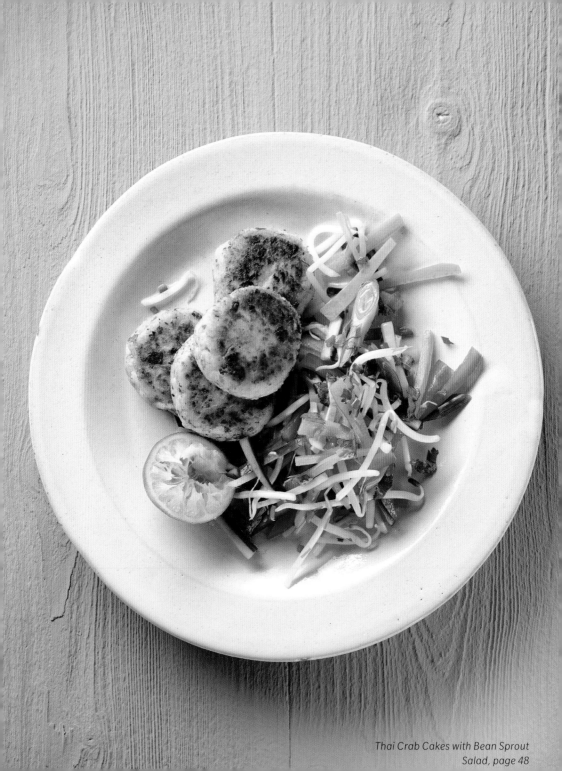

Thai Crab Cakes with Bean Sprout Salad, page 48

Go light

(light meals & lunches)

GREEN RECIPES (MAX 300 KCALS)	AMBER RECIPES (MAX 350 KCALS)

Fresh mussel and tomato soup

Aromatic Thai prawn broth

Squash and butterbean soup

Tuscan bean and vegetable soup with cavolo nero

Indian spiced lentil soup with tarka garnish

Tofu kebabs with garlic pak choi

Thai crab cakes with bean sprout salad

Chicory, pear and chickpea salad

Vietnamese chicken salad

Thai chicken lettuce 'parcels'

Quick summer chicken with minted peas

Griddled chicken and squash salad

Barbecued California salad with grilled shrimp

Cheat's cauliflower 'rice' salad

Cheat's falafels with garlic yoghurt skordalia

Cheat's chicken burgers with tzatziki

Spicy chicken noodle soup

Sushi and Japanese salad

Cheat's loaded potato skins with variation

Chilli baked sweet potatoes

Fruity quinoa salad with roasted vegetables

Cheat's quick 'n' easy pizzas

Cheat's beans on toast

Cheat's tuna melt 'toasties'

Cheat's crispy chicken nuggets

Cheat's chicken Caesar salad

Cheat's hamburgers

Cheat's steak 'sandwich'

Cheat's crunchy fish fingers

Cheesy chicken quesadillas *with variation*

FRESH MUSSEL
and TOMATO SOUP

This Mediterranean-style soup is really healthy and surprisingly filling. Mussels are economical, a good source of protein and cook very quickly. It's important to follow the guidelines on preparing them and to throw away any that are open before cooking or fail to open afterwards. Try adding chopped basil or coriander instead of parsley, or add a few saffron threads to the soup – the calories will stay the same.

SERVES 4

Prep: 20 minutes

Cook: 35–40 minutes

Per serving:

300 kcals

1255 kJ

7.5g fat

Low GI

1kg/2lb 2oz live mussels

low-cal spray oil

1 large red onion, finely chopped

1 large leek, chopped

2 garlic cloves, crushed

1 red chilli, deseeded and diced (optional)

1 tsp smoked paprika

2 x 400g/14oz (3½ cups) cans chopped tomatoes

600ml/1 pint (2½ cups) fish or vegetable stock

sea salt and freshly ground black pepper

a handful of parsley, chopped

1 Put the mussels in a large bowl of cold water and discard any that are open or cracked. Scrub the rest under cold running water and scrape away the wispy 'beards'.

2 Lightly spray a large saucepan with oil and cook the onion, leek, garlic and chilli (if using) over a low heat for 8–10 minutes, stirring occasionally, until softened. Stir in the paprika.

3 Add the tomatoes and stock, then bring to the boil. Cook vigorously for 1 minute, then reduce the heat, cover the pan and cook gently for 10–15 minutes.

4 Meanwhile, cook the mussels. Tip them into a large heavy-based saucepan, add a tablespoon of water and cover with a lid. Place over a high heat and cook, shaking gently from time to time, for about 3 minutes, or until the shells open. Drain in a colander placed over a bowl to catch any juices. Throw away any mussels that have failed to open.

5 Strain the mussel juice through a sieve and add to the soup. Remove about three-quarters of the mussels from their shells (reserve the rest for the garnish) and stir them gently into the soup. Season to taste with salt and pepper, and simmer gently for 5 minutes. Stir in the parsley.

6 Ladle the soup into 4 deep serving bowls and add the reserved mussels in their shells. Serve immediately.

Amber option: For extra flavour, stir 1 tsp green pesto into each bowl of soup. This will add 23 kcals and 2.2g fat per serving.

AROMATIC THAI PRAWN BROTH

This spicy clear seafood broth takes less than 25 minutes to make from start to finish. There's enough soup for four people, but you can freeze two or three portions or store overnight in an airtight container in the fridge. Instead of prawns (shrimp) you can stir-fry 400g/14oz thinly sliced chicken breast fillets with the spring onions (scallions) and mushrooms until golden brown. The calories will remain the same.

SERVES 4

Prep: 10 minutes

Cook: 15 minutes

Per serving:

200 kcals

837 kJ

3.6g fat

Low GI

low-cal spray oil

8 spring onions (scallions), sliced

2 garlic cloves, finely sliced

2.5cm/1in fresh root ginger, peeled and diced

1 red chilli, cut into fine shreds

200g/7oz mushrooms, thinly sliced

1.2 litres/2 pints (5 cups) hot vegetable stock

1 lemongrass stalk, peeled and bashed with a rolling pin

2 fresh (or dried) kaffir lime leaves

200g/7oz spring greens or spinach, shredded

450g/1lb large raw tiger prawns (jumbo shrimp)

200g/7oz (2 cups) bean sprouts

1 tbsp dark soy sauce

1 tbsp nam pla (Thai fish sauce)

juice of 1 lime

1 small bunch of fresh coriander (cilantro), chopped

1 Lightly spray a large saucepan with oil and set over a medium heat. When it's hot, add the spring onions, garlic, ginger, chilli and mushrooms. Stir-fry for 2–3 minutes until the vegetables start to colour.

2 Add the hot stock, lemongrass and kaffir lime leaves and bring to the boil. Reduce the heat and simmer gently for 5 minutes.

3 Add the spring greens or spinach and prawns and simmer for 4–5 minutes, or until the prawns turn uniformly pink and the greens wilt a little but still retain some bite.

4 Stir in the bean sprouts, soy sauce, nam pla and lime juice. Remove and discard the lemongrass stalk. Add the coriander and ladle into shallow serving bowls. Serve immediately.

> **TIP:** If you don't like coriander, try mint or Thai basil instead.

SQUASH *and* BUTTERBEAN SOUP

This gently spiced golden soup is not only warming but surprisingly filling too. For more heat, add a pinch of dried chilli flakes or even a diced fresh chilli. You can substitute cannellini beans for the butterbeans (lima beans).

SERVES: 4

Prep: 10 minutes

Cook: 35 minutes

Per serving:

245 kcals

1025 kJ

1.8g fat

Low GI

low-cal spray oil

1 onion, finely chopped

2 garlic cloves, crushed

900g/2lb butternut squash, peeled, deseeded and cubed

1 tsp ground cumin

½ tsp ground nutmeg

½ tsp ground turmeric

1.2 litres/2 pints (5 cups) vegetable stock

1 x 400g/14oz (4 cups) can butterbeans (lima beans), rinsed and drained

sea salt and freshly ground black pepper

4 tbsp 0% fat Greek yoghurt

a small handful of parsley, chopped

1 Spray a large saucepan lightly with oil and set over a low heat. Add the onion and garlic and cook for about 5 minutes until the onion starts to soften. Add the squash and cook for 5 minutes, stirring occasionally. Stir in the ground spices and cook for 1 minute.

2 Add the vegetable stock and bring to the boil. Reduce the heat to a simmer and cook gently for 15 minutes until the squash is tender. Add half the butterbeans to the soup.

3 Pour the soup, in batches, into a blender or food processor and blitz until thick and smooth. Alternatively, use an electric hand blender.

4 Pour the soup back into the pan and stir in the remaining butterbeans. Season to taste with salt and pepper and heat through gently.

5 Serve the hot soup in bowls, topped with a swirl of yoghurt and sprinkled with parsley.

TUSCAN BEAN *and* VEGETABLE SOUP *with* CAVOLO NERO

This soup is infinitely versatile and you can vary the vegetables according to the season and what's in the fridge. For instance, swap the fennel for some celery, or the cavolo nero for kale, spinach or spring greens. Cavolo nero is a slightly bitter-tasting Italian cabbage with blackish green leaves, and is a wonderful source of vitamins and minerals.

SERVES 4

Prep: 15 minutes

Cook: 40 minutes

Per serving:

295 kcals

1234 kJ

3.3g fat

Low GI

low-cal spray oil

1 onion, chopped

1 leek, cleaned, trimmed and chopped

1 small fennel bulb, halved and thinly sliced

2 carrots, diced

2 garlic cloves, crushed

900ml/1½ pints (3¾ cups) vegetable stock

450g/1lb ripe tomatoes, coarsely chopped

stripped leaves of 2 sprigs of thyme

stripped and chopped leaves of 1 sprig of rosemary

2 x 400g/14oz (4 cups) cans cannellini beans, rinsed and drained

200g/7oz cavolo nero, cut into small wedges or shredded

sea salt and freshly ground black pepper

1 Lightly spray a large saucepan with oil and set over a low to medium heat. Cook the onion, leek, fennel and carrots, stirring occasionally, for 8–10 minutes until softened but not coloured. Add the garlic and cook for 1 minute.

2 Add the stock and tomatoes and bring to the boil. Reduce the heat to a simmer, add the thyme and rosemary and cook gently for 40 minutes or until all the vegetables are cooked and tender.

3 Add the beans and cavolo nero and simmer for 3–4 minutes – just long enough for the cavolo to wilt without losing its texture and colour. Season to taste with salt and pepper.

4 Ladle the hot soup into shallow bowls and serve immediately.

> **TIP:** You can use canned chopped tomatoes instead of fresh – the calories will stay the same.

INDIAN SPICED LENTIL SOUP *with* TARKA GARNISH

Here's a really healthy and nutritious soup to warm you up on a cold day. Use the small red lentils, not the larger brown or Puy ones, as they will soften, thicken and colour the soup. They are a good source of protein, vitamins B1 and B6, minerals and fibre.

SERVES 4

Prep: 15 minutes

Cook: 40 minutes

Per serving:

240 kcals

1004 kJ

2.2g fat

Low GI

low-cal spray oil

1 onion, finely chopped

2 celery sticks, diced

2 carrots, diced

2 garlic cloves, crushed

2.5cm/1in fresh root ginger, peeled and diced

1 tsp ground cumin

1 tsp ground turmeric

½ tsp chilli powder

200g/7oz (1 cup) split red lentils

1.2 litres/2 pints (5 cups) vegetable stock

juice of ½ lemon

sea salt and freshly ground black pepper

a handful of coriander (cilantro), chopped

4 tbsp 0% fat Greek yoghurt

For the tarka garnish:

low-cal spray oil

1 small red onion, thinly sliced

1 red chilli, deseeded and cut into fine shreds

1 tsp black mustard seeds

1 tsp cumin seeds

1 Spray a large saucepan lightly with oil and set over a medium heat. Add the onion, celery, carrots, garlic and ginger and cook, stirring occasionally, for about 5 minutes until starting to soften. Stir in the spices and lentils and cook for 1 minute.

2 Add the vegetable stock and bring to the boil. Reduce the heat and simmer gently for about 25 minutes until the vegetables are tender and the lentils have broken down to thicken the soup.

3 Use an electric hand blender to purée the soup or blitz in batches in a blender and return to the pan. Add the lemon juice and season to taste with salt and pepper. Heat through gently, then stir in the coriander.

4 Meanwhile, make the tarka topping: lightly spray a small frying pan (skillet) with oil and set over a medium heat. Cook the onion, stirring occasionally, until tender, golden and starting to crisp on the edges. Add the chilli and seeds and cook for 1 minute until the mustard seeds start to pop. Remove from the heat immediately.

5 Ladle the hot soup into bowls and swirl in the yoghurt. Sprinkle with the tarka and serve immediately.

TOFU KEBABS *with* GARLIC PAK CHOI

With its silky texture and high protein content, tofu (bean curd) is a very healthy food. Delicately flavoured, it benefits from being marinated in flavoursome and spicy marinades before cooking.

SERVES 2

Prep: 10 minutes

Marinate: 10 mins

Cook: 5–10 minutes

Per serving:

240 kcals

1004 kJ

8g fat

Low GI

2 tbsp soy sauce

2 tsp tomato paste

1 garlic clove, crushed

200g/7oz tofu (bean curd), cut into cubes

1 yellow (bell) pepper, deseeded and cut into chunks

1 red (bell) pepper, deseeded and cut into chunks

1 courgette (zucchini), cut into chunks

1 red onion, peeled and cut into wedges

low-cal spray oil

For the crispy garlic pak choi:

200g/7oz pak choi (bok choy)

low-cal spray oil

2 garlic cloves, thinly sliced

2.5cm/1in fresh root ginger, peeled and cut into thin matchsticks

1 red chilli, deseeded and cut into fine shreds

balsamic vinegar for drizzling (optional)

1 Mix together the soy sauce, tomato paste and garlic in a bowl. Add the tofu cubes and turn in the marinade to coat them. Leave to marinate for 10 minutes.

2 Thread the tofu, peppers, courgette and red onion alternately onto 2 long or 4 short skewers and spray them lightly with oil. Cook on a hot griddle pan or barbecue or under a preheated grill (broiler) for about 5 minutes, turning them occasionally, until the vegetables are tender and slightly charred on the edges.

3 Meanwhile, cut the pak choi in half lengthways, and then cut each half into chunky wedges. Cook in a steamer (or colander) set over a pan of boiling water for 4–5 minutes until just tender.

4 Lightly spray a small frying pan (skillet) with oil and set over a high heat. When it's smoking hot, add the garlic, ginger and chilli and stir-fry for 1–2 minutes until the garlic is crispy and golden but not browned. Watch carefully to prevent it burning.

5 Arrange the tofu kebabs on 2 serving plates. Serve immediately with the steamed pak choi topped with the crispy garlic mixture and drizzled with balsamic if you like.

THAI CRAB CAKES *with* BEAN SPROUT SALAD

For the best results use fresh crabmeat, but if it's not available frozen or canned is fine. When buying mayonnaise, always choose extra light. There are only 10 kcals and 0.5g fat per tablespoon versus 35 kcals and 4g fat in the same amount of light mayonnaise.

SERVES 2

Prep: 20 minutes

Chill: 15–30 mins

Cook: 4–6 minutes

Per serving:

250 kcals

1046 kJ

3.4g fat

Low GI

300g/10oz fresh white crabmeat

1 red chilli, diced

4 spring onions (scallions), finely chopped

2 garlic cloves, crushed

a large handful of coriander (cilantro)

2 tsp nam pla (Thai fish sauce)

1 tbsp extra light mayonnaise

flour for dusting

low-cal spray oil

For the bean sprout salad:

200g/7oz (2 cups) bean sprouts

¼ small cucumber, cut into matchstick strips

1 carrot, peeled and cut into matchstick strips

1 red or yellow (bell) pepper, deseeded and thinly sliced

3 spring onions (scallions), chopped

2 tbsp chopped fresh coriander (cilantro)

1 red chilli, cut into fine shreds

2 tbsp nam pla (Thai fish sauce)

juice of 1 lime

liquid artificial sweetener, e.g. stevia, to taste

1 Put the crabmeat, diced chilli, spring onions, garlic, coriander, nam pla and mayonnaise in a blender or food processor and blitz until you have a thick sludge.

2 Divide the mixture into 8 portions and shape with your hands into little patties. Dust them very lightly with flour and chill in the fridge for 15–30 minutes to firm them up.

3 Make the bean sprout salad: in a bowl, mix together the bean sprouts, cucumber, carrot, pepper, spring onions and coriander. Put the chilli, nam pla and lime juice in a smaller bowl and mix well. Add a few drops of artificial sweetener to taste. Pour over the salad and toss gently.

4 Lightly spray a frying pan (skillet) with oil and set over a medium to high heat. When the pan is hot, add the crab cakes and cook for about 2–3 minutes each side, until golden brown. Take care when you turn them over – use a spatula and do it gently to keep their shape. Serve immediately with the bean sprout salad.

> **TIP:** If wished, add some shredded Chinese cabbage, sliced radishes or fennel to the salad. The extra calories will be negligible.

Amber option: If you can't bear eating crab cakes without sweet chilli sauce, remember that every tablespoon adds a whopping 35 kcals.

CHICORY, PEAR and CHICKPEA SALAD

This is a great winter salad – crisp and filling – and it goes well with some cold chicken or turkey. If wished, you can substitute a diced crunchy apple for the pear.

SERVES 2

Prep: 15 minutes

Per serving:

300 kcals

1255 kJ

5.6g fat

Low GI

1 head chicory (Belgian endive)

1 head radicchio or red chicory

¼ red onion, finely chopped

2 spring onions (scallions), finely chopped

200g/7oz (generous 1 cup) canned chickpeas, rinsed and drained

1 small bunch of parsley, chopped

3 tbsp oil-free lemon vinaigrette (see page 53)

sea salt and freshly ground black pepper

200g/7oz (scant 1 cup) low-fat cottage cheese

1 ripe medium pear, halved, cored and thinly sliced

1 Trim the ends off the chicory and thinly slice into rounds. Separate the radicchio into leaves.

2 Mix the chicory, radicchio, red onion, spring onions, chickpeas and parsley in a serving bowl. Sprinkle the vinaigrette over the top and toss gently. Season to taste with salt and pepper and toss again gently.

3 Divide the salad between 2 serving plates and top with the cottage cheese and sliced pear. Serve immediately.

Amber option: Dice the flesh of ½ small avocado and mix into the salad. This adds 40 kcals and 4g fat per serving.

VIETNAMESE CHICKEN SALAD

This crunchy salad makes a great light meal. It's also a really good way to use up leftover cooked chicken or turkey. The thinner the strips of carrot, courgette (zucchini) and cucumber, the better – a spiraliser gives the best results if you have one, or just use a potato peeler.

SERVES 2

Prep: 20 minutes

Cook: 6–8 minutes

Per serving:

250 kcals

1046 kJ

3g fat

Low GI

1 carrot, cut into thin strips

1 courgette (zucchini), cut into long, thin strips

85g/3oz mange tout (snow peas), trimmed and halved lengthways

4 spring onions (scallions), thinly sliced

¼ cucumber, cut into thin strips

1 Little Gem lettuce, leaves separated

low-cal spray oil

½ red onion, thinly sliced

2 x 125g/4oz skinned chicken breast fillets, cut into thin strips

a few basil leaves, chopped

a handful of coriander (cilantro), chopped

lime wedges, to serve

For the dressing:

1 Thai red chilli, deseeded and cut into fine shreds

2 garlic cloves, thinly sliced

2 tbsp nam pla (Thai fish sauce)

1 tbsp water or rice vinegar

juice of 1 lime

liquid artificial sweetener, e.g. stevia, to taste (optional)

1 Mix together the carrot, courgette, mange tout, spring onions, cucumber and lettuce in a large bowl.

2 Lightly spray a non-stick frying pan (skillet) with oil and set over a medium heat. Cook the red onion and chicken for 6–8 minutes, turning occasionally, until the onion is just tender and the chicken is cooked through and golden brown.

3 Meanwhile, mix all the dressing ingredients together in a small bowl and gently toss most of it through the salad vegetables, reserving some to finish.

4 Divide the salad between 2 serving plates and top with the warm chicken strips and red onion. Sprinkle with the basil and coriander and drizzle the remaining dressing over the top. Serve immediately with lime wedges.

Amber option: For a more substantial dinner, add 60g/2oz rice noodles (dry weight). Prepare as per the instructions on the packet and toss with the salad. This will add 113 kcals per serving.

THAI CHICKEN LETTUCE 'PARCELS'

This fresh, zingy salad is bursting with Thai flavours and perfectly complements the spicy chicken. You can buy ready minced (ground) chicken or just process some skinned chicken breast fillets in a food processor.

SERVES 2

Prep: 15 minutes

Cook: 10–12 mins

Per serving:

270 kcals

1130 kJ

4g fat

Low GI

1 lemongrass stalk, peeled and chopped

2 garlic cloves, crushed

2 tsp grated fresh root ginger

1 red chilli, deseeded and diced

low-cal spray oil

250g/9oz (generous 1 cup) minced (ground) lean chicken breast

4 spring onions (scallions), chopped

175g/6oz spring greens, spinach or kale, shredded

1 tbsp nam pla (Thai fish sauce)

1–2 tbsp water

juice of ½ lime

4 large iceberg lettuce leaves

For the crunchy salad:

100g/3½oz (1 cup) bean sprouts

1 carrot, peeled and cut into thin matchsticks

¼ cucumber, cut into matchsticks

2 spring onions (scallions), sliced

1 red chilli, deseeded and cut into fine shreds

1 small bunch of mint or coriander (cilantro)

1 small bunch of basil

1 tbsp nam pla (Thai fish sauce)

juice of ½ lime

liquid artificial sweetener, e.g. stevia, to taste

1 Put the lemongrass, garlic, ginger and chilli in a blender or food processor and blitz to a paste.

2 Make the crunchy salad: put the bean sprouts, carrot, cucumber, spring onions and chilli in a bowl. Strip the leaves off the herb stalks and add. In a small bowl, mix the nam pla and lime juice with sweetener to taste.

3 Lightly spray a wok or non-stick frying pan (skillet) with oil and set over a high heat. Add the blitzed spicy lemongrass mixture and cook, stirring, for 1 minute. Add the chicken and stir-fry for 3–4 minutes until browned all over.

4 Add the spring onions and greens and stir-fry for 2 minutes. Stir in the nam pla and enough of the water to moisten the mixture. Reduce the heat and cook gently for 4–5 minutes.

5 Add the lime juice and divide the mixture between the lettuce leaves. Fold over and roll up to make 4 parcels. Place 2 on each serving plate.

6 Toss the crunchy salad in the dressing and serve immediately with the chicken parcels.

Amber options: Stir 25g/1oz cashew nuts into the chicken mixture and you'll add 73 kcals and 6g fat per serving! Serve each portion drizzled with 1 tsp sweet chilli sauce and you'll have an extra 12 kcals.

QUICK SUMMER CHICKEN *with* MINTED PEAS

SERVES 2

Prep: 10 minutes

Cook: 35 minutes

Per serving:

280 kcals

1172 kJ

3.5g fat

Low GI

This is a healthy light meal for a warm day. If you don't have fresh peas, use frozen ones instead. We've suggested green beans and baby carrots as a vegetable accompaniment but you could make a green salad of Little Gem lettuce leaves, cucumber, spring onions (scallions) and fresh herbs tossed in an oil-free vinaigrette, and save about 30 kcals per serving.

low-cal spray oil

1 onion, finely chopped

1 garlic clove, crushed

2 x 125g/4oz skinned, boned chicken breasts

180ml/6fl oz (¾ cup) hot chicken stock

150g/5oz (scant 1 cup) fresh shelled peas

2 tbsp 0% fat Greek yoghurt

grated zest of 1 lemon

a handful of mint, finely chopped

a squeeze of lemon juice

sea salt and freshly ground black pepper

150g/5oz fine green beans, trimmed

150g/5oz baby carrots, trimmed

1 Lightly spray a frying pan (skillet) with oil and set over a low to medium heat. Cook the onion and garlic, stirring occasionally, for 6–8 minutes until softened. Add the chicken and cook for 4 minutes each side until coloured.

2 Pour in the hot stock and simmer gently over a low heat for 10 minutes, turning the chicken halfway through.

3 Add the peas and simmer for about 5 minutes until tender. If the chicken is cooked through, take the pan off the heat and stir in the yoghurt, lemon zest and mint. Season to taste with a squeeze of lemon juice and some salt and pepper.

4 Meanwhile, cook the green beans and carrots in a pan of boiling salted water or a steamer until just tender. Drain well.

5 Serve the chicken and peas in the creamy sauce with the beans and carrots.

GRIDDLED CHICKEN
and SQUASH SALAD

This delicious salad is best eaten warm. It's very versatile and you can change some of the ingredients without changing the overall calorie count: swap the squash for pumpkin or the rocket (arugula) for baby spinach or watercress. The vinaigrette dressing is made without oil and sweetened with stevia, a zero-calorie natural sweetener extracted from the leaves of a plant.

SERVES 2

Prep: 20 minutes

Cook: 25–35 mins

Per serving:

290 kcals

1213 kJ

5g fat

Low GI

1 tsp coriander seeds

2 tsp cumin seeds

200g/7oz butternut squash, halved, deseeded and cut into strips

1 red onion, cut into wedges

low-cal spray oil

sea salt crystals and freshly ground black pepper

2 x 125g/4oz skinned, boned chicken breasts

60g/2oz wild rocket (arugula)

seeds of 1 small pomegranate

balsamic vinegar for drizzling

For the oil-free lemon vinaigrette:

1 garlic clove, crushed

1 tsp grated fresh root ginger

1 tsp Dijon mustard

juice of 1 lemon

2 tbsp water

1 tsp poppy seeds

liquid stevia, to taste

1 Preheat the oven to 200°C, 400°F, gas mark 6.

2 With a pestle and mortar, coarsely grind the coriander and cumin seeds.

3 Place the squash and red onion in a roasting pan and sprinkle the ground seeds over the top. Lightly spray with oil and season with salt and pepper. Roast in the preheated oven for 25–35 minutes, turning the vegetables once or twice, until tender and golden brown.

4 Meanwhile, lightly spray a ridged griddle pan with oil and set over a medium heat. Add the chicken breasts and cook for about 15 minutes, turning occasionally, until cooked right through, golden brown and attractively striped.

5 Make the lemon vinaigrette: put all the ingredients except the stevia in a small blender and blitz until well blended. Sweeten to taste with the stevia. Alternatively, whisk everything together.

6 Put the roasted squash, rocket and most of the pomegranate seeds in a bowl and toss lightly in the vinaigrette. Divide between 2 serving plates or shallow bowls.

7 Slice the warm chicken breasts with a very sharp knife and arrange on top of the salad. Drizzle with balsamic vinegar and scatter with the remaining pomegranate seeds. Serve immediately.

BARBECUED CALIFORNIA SALAD *with* GRILLED SHRIMP

Barbecued salads are very popular in California where all the salad leaves and vegetables are thrown onto the hot grill until they are just tender but still retain a little bite. We've added juicy prawns (shrimp) but you could use 200g/7oz chicken fillets or tofu (bean curd) instead and the calories will stay the same.

SERVES 2

Prep: 15 minutes

Cook: 15 minutes

Per serving:

290 kcals

1213 kJ

3.4g fat

Low GI

---

low-cal spray oil

150g/5oz thin asparagus, trimmed

200g/7oz courgettes (zucchini), sliced lengthways

8 baby leeks, trimmed

1 head radicchio, separated into leaves

125g/4oz leafy greens, e.g. kale or Swiss chard

3 tbsp oil-free lemon vinaigrette (see page 53)

sea salt and freshly ground black pepper

300g/10oz raw king prawns (jumbo shrimp)

juice of ½ lime

balsamic vinegar for drizzling

a small handful of coriander (cilantro), chopped

For the spicy yoghurt:

125g/4oz (½ cup) 0% fat Greek yoghurt

a good pinch of curry powder or garam masala

1 Preheat a barbecue or large non-stick griddle pan. It must get really hot before you start cooking. Spray lightly with oil.

2 Cook the asparagus, courgettes and leeks, turning them occasionally, for 5–7 minutes, until just tender and slightly charred. Remove as they become ready and keep warm – you can cook them in batches if wished.

3 Add the radicchio and greens and grill (broil) for about 2–3 minutes, until they start to char. Remove and tear into large pieces. Place them in a bowl with the grilled vegetables. Toss gently in the lemon vinaigrette and check the seasoning.

4 Add the prawns to the barbecue or griddle pan and cook for 2 minutes, turning them over as soon as they turn pink underneath and removing from the barbecue or pan when they are uniformly pink.

5 Divide the salad between 2 serving plates and top with the prawns. Sprinkle with the lime juice and drizzle with balsamic vinegar.

6 Mix the yoghurt with the ground spice and add a little black pepper. Serve with the salad, sprinkled with coriander.

CHEAT'S CAULIFLOWER 'RICE' SALAD

SERVES 2

Prep: 15 minutes

Cook: 35 minute

Per serving:

300 kcals

1255 kJ

5.9g fat

Low GI

Cauliflower 'rice' is really healthy and slimming – a great diet 'cheat' and an effective way to reduce your carb intake. It sounds complicated but nothing could be easier – just blitz the cauliflower in a food processor and then warm through gently with some seeds, spices or herbs.

450g/1lb peeled butternut squash, deseeded and cubed

low-cal spray oil

sea salt and freshly ground black pepper

200g/7oz (generous 1 cup) canned chickpeas, rinsed and drained

grated zest of ½ lemon

a good pinch of chilli powder

1 small cauliflower, quartered and core removed

2 garlic cloves, crushed

1 tbsp black mustard seeds

a pinch of dried chilli flakes

2 tsp cumin seeds

85g/3oz wild rocket (arugula)

4 spring onions (scallions), finely sliced

100g/3½oz cherry or baby plum tomatoes, quartered

a handful of mint or flat-leaf parsley, chopped

juice of 1 lemon

4 tbsp 0% fat Greek yoghurt

1 Preheat the oven to 180°C, 350°F, gas mark 4.

2 Arrange the squash in a large baking tin (pan) and spray lightly with oil. Grind over some salt and pepper and roast in the preheated oven for 25–30 minutes until tender.

3 Meanwhile, put the chickpeas on a baking tray (cookie sheet) lined with baking parchment. Sprinkle over the lemon zest, chilli powder and some salt and pepper and spray lightly with oil. Roast in the oven for 15–20 minutes until crisp and golden brown. Remove and cool.

4 Cut the cauliflower into small florets or chop into smaller pieces. Pulse them several times in a food processor until they have the consistency of grains of rice.

5 Lightly spray a large frying pan (skillet) with oil and set over a low to medium heat. Cook the garlic and mustard seeds for 2 minutes, then add the chilli flakes, cumin seeds and cauliflower and cook for 3–5 minutes, stirring well, until the cauliflower is warm and crunchy.

6 Transfer to a large serving bowl with the rocket, spring onions, tomatoes and herbs. Add the roasted vegetables and toss gently. Drizzle with the lemon juice and check the seasoning. Serve topped with a dollop of Greek yoghurt.

CHEAT'S FALAFELS *with* GARLIC YOGHURT SKORDALIA

These lovely green-flecked falafels are high in protein and dietary fibre but low in calories. They're quick and easy to make and then wrapped in iceberg lettuce leaves with a really garlicky cheat on skordalia, which is usually made with potatoes and oil.

SERVES 2

Prep: 15 minutes

Cook: 15–20 mins

Per serving:

300 kcals

1255 kJ

7g fat

Low GI

low-cal spray oil

1 small onion, finely chopped

1 garlic clove, crushed

400g/14oz (generous 2 cups) canned chickpeas, rinsed and drained

1 tsp ground cumin

1 large bunch of coriander (cilantro), chopped

a good squeeze of lemon juice

sea salt and freshly ground black pepper

1 small free-range egg, beaten

4 large iceberg lettuce leaves

cayenne or paprika for dusting

For the garlic yoghurt skordalia:

100g/3½oz (scant ½ cup) 0% fat Greek yoghurt

3 garlic cloves, crushed

2 tsp lemon juice

2 tbsp finely chopped mint (or 1 tbsp dried)

1 Lightly spray a saucepan with oil and set over a low heat. Add the onion and garlic to the hot pan and cook gently, stirring occasionally, for 6–8 minutes until softened.

2 Mash the chickpeas coarsely with a potato masher and mix in the cooked onion mixture, the cumin, coriander, lemon juice and salt and pepper to taste. Add enough beaten egg to bind the mixture together. Alternatively, if you prefer a smoother, less grainy texture, you can blitz everything briefly in a blender.

3 Divide the mixture into 8 portions and use your hands to shape each one into a small ball.

4 Lightly spray a non-stick frying pan (skillet) with oil and set over a medium heat. Add the falafels to the hot pan and cook for about 5 minutes, turning them occasionally, until cooked and golden brown all over. (Alternatively, you can bake them in the oven at 200°C, 400°F, gas mark 6 for 10 minutes.)

5 Meanwhile, to make the garlic skordalia, mix all the ingredients together in a bowl.

6 Divide the falafels between the iceberg lettuce leaves and top with the garlic skordalia. Dust with cayenne pepper or paprika and fold over or roll up to make 'wraps'. Eat warm or cold.

Amber option: If you divide the falafels and skordalia between 2 plain wraps, you will add between 100 and 200 kcals per serving! Check the label carefully.

CHEAT'S CHICKEN BURGERS *with* TZATZIKI

Substituting aubergine (eggplant) slices for burger buns reduces the calories, eliminates the carbs and tastes delicious. These succulent chicken burgers are flavoured with hot and spicy harissa paste and served with tzatziki.

....

SERVES 2

Prep: 20 minutes

Chill: 15 minutes

Cook: 16 minutes

Per serving:

250 kcals

1046 kJ

2.5g fat

Low GI

250g/9oz minced (ground) lean chicken

½ red onion, diced

2 garlic cloves, crushed

½ tsp ground cumin

grated zest of 1 small lemon

a small handful of coriander (cilantro), chopped

2 tsp tomato paste

a squeeze of harissa paste

sea salt and freshly ground black pepper

flour for dusting

1 small aubergine (eggplant), trimmed and cut into 4 thick round slices

low-cal spray oil

For the tzatziki:

120g/4oz (½ cup) 0% fat Greek yoghurt

1 garlic clove, crushed

¼ small cucumber, diced

1 small bunch of mint or coriander (cilantro), finely chopped

juice of ½ small lemon

1 Preheat the oven to 200°C, 400°F, gas mark 6.

2 Mix the chicken, red onion, garlic, cumin, lemon zest and coriander in a bowl. Stir in the tomato paste and add a dash of harissa – not too much as it's very fiery. Season lightly.

3 Divide the mixture into 2 equal-sized portions and, with lightly floured hands, shape into burgers. Cover and chill in the fridge for at least 15 minutes to firm them up.

4 Meanwhile, make the tzatziki: mix all the ingredients together in a bowl and season to taste with salt and pepper.

5 Place the aubergine slices on a baking tray (cookie sheet) lined with foil and spray lightly with oil. Season with a little salt and pepper. Bake in the preheated oven for 7–8 minutes, then turn them over and cook for another 7–8 minutes until golden brown and starting to crisp.

6 At the same time, cook the burgers in an oiled griddle pan or under a preheated hot grill (broiler) for 6–8 minutes each side, until cooked all the way through and golden brown.

7 To serve, place a baked aubergine slice on each serving plate and top with a chicken burger and a spoonful of tzatziki. Cover with another aubergine slice and serve immediately with the remaining tzatziki and a green salad.

SPICY CHICKEN NOODLE SOUP

Nutritionally, this is a complete meal-in-a-bowl. There's enough soup for four people, but you can cool and freeze two or three portions if you wish, or store in an airtight container in the fridge overnight. If you don't like coriander (cilantro) use fresh basil or mint instead to make the curry paste.

SERVES 4

Prep: 15 minutes

Cook: 15 minutes

Per serving:

350 kcals

1464 kJ

9.2g fat

Medium GI

1 green chilli

2 lemongrass stalks, peeled and chopped

2 garlic cloves, peeled

1 tsp grated fresh root ginger

grated zest and juice of 1 lime

1 bunch of fresh coriander (cilantro)

100g/3½oz thin rice noodles (dry weight)

low-cal spray oil

1 bunch of spring onions (scallions), thickly sliced

450g/1lb skinned chicken breast fillets, sliced

1 tsp crushed coriander seeds

960ml/32fl oz (4 cups) hot chicken stock

210ml/7fl oz (scant 1 cup) canned reduced-fat coconut milk

1 tbsp nam pla (Thai fish sauce)

2 kaffir lime leaves, finely shredded (optional)

200g/7oz baby spinach leaves

1 red bird's eye chilli, deseeded and cut into fine shreds

1 Put the green chilli, lemongrass, garlic, ginger, lime zest and coriander (keep a few leaves to serve) in a food processor or blender. Blitz to a thick green paste.

2 Put the rice noodles in a large, shallow heatproof bowl and cover with boiling water. Set aside to soak for 10 minutes, stirring occasionally to prevent the noodles sticking together. Or follow the instructions on the packet.

3 Meanwhile, lightly spray a large saucepan with oil and set over a medium heat. Add the spring onions and cook for 1 minute. Turn up the heat and add the chicken. Stir-fry for 3–4 minutes until golden brown on both sides.

4 Stir in the green paste and crushed coriander seeds and cook for 1 minute, then add the hot chicken stock, coconut milk, nam pla and kaffir lime leaves (if using). Simmer for 5 minutes or until the chicken is cooked through. Stir in the lime juice and spinach, and cook for 1 more minute – just long enough for the spinach to wilt and turn bright green.

5 Drain the rice noodles and divide between 4 shallow serving bowls. Pour the soup over the top and sprinkle with the reserved coriander and chilli. Serve immediately.

SUSHI *and* JAPANESE SALAD

Sushi is surprisingly simple to make yourself at home. You can now buy all the ingredients – special sushi rice, mirin, nori and wasabi – in most supermarkets. We've served ours with a delicious crunchy Japanese salad.

SERVES 2

Prep: 30 minutes

Chill: 15 minutes

Per serving:

350 kcals

1464 kJ

7.5g fat

Medium GI

100g/3½oz (scant ½ cup) sushi rice (dry weight)

1 tbsp rice vinegar

1 tsp mirin

¼ cucumber

2 sheets of nori seaweed

60g/2oz thinly sliced smoked salmon, cut into long strips

1 tsp wasabi paste

a small handful of chives

Japanese soy sauce for sprinkling or dipping

For the Japanese salad:

100g/3½oz frozen edamame beans, defrosted

1 carrot, peeled and cut into long, thin matchsticks

2 spring onions (scallions), cut into long, thin strips

8 radishes, thinly sliced

2 tbsp Japanese soy sauce

1 tbsp rice vinegar

juice of ½ lime

1 garlic clove, crushed (optional)

a few drops of liquid artificial sweetener, e.g. stevia

2 tsp black or white sesame seeds

1 Cook the rice according to the directions on the packet – it will take about 10–15 minutes. Stir the rice vinegar and mirin into the cooked rice, then cover the pan and leave until the rice is at room temperature.

2 Meanwhile, peel the cucumber, then cut it in half lengthways and scoop out the seeds. Cut each cucumber half into long, thin strips.

3 Place the nori sheets, shiny side down, on a bamboo sushi mat or a work surface covered with cling film (plastic wrap). Divide the rice between the sheets, spreading it out evenly and level, leaving a 1cm/½in border along the long edges.

4 Place the smoked salmon on top of the rice and dot with the wasabi paste. Top with the cucumber strips and chives. Using the cling film and sushi mat (if using one) to help you, lift the long bottom edge of each nori sheet over the rice and smoked salmon filling and roll up towards the top, pressing down firmly as you go. When you get to the top, brush lightly with a little water to seal it.

5 Put the 2 rolls in the fridge and leave to chill for at least 15 minutes or until you're ready to serve.

6 While the sushi rolls are chilling, make the Japanese salad. In a bowl, mix together the edamame beans, carrot, spring onions and radishes. Put the soy sauce, vinegar, lime juice and garlic (if using) in a small bowl and beat together. Sweeten to taste with artificial sweetener and stir in the sesame seeds. Lightly toss the salad in the dressing.

7 To serve, slice each sushi roll into 6 rounds. Serve with the Japanese salad and some soy sauce.

CHEAT'S LOADED POTATO SKINS

These loaded potato skins make delicious hot snacks.
You can speed up the baking time by cooking the potatoes
in a microwave. Vegetarians can omit the ham and add
another tablespoon of grated cheese.

SERVES 2

Prep: 5 minutes

Cook: 25–30 mins

Per serving:

100 kcals

418 kJ

1.4g fat

High GI

2 x 75g/3oz small potatoes

low-cal spray oil

sea salt crystals

For the cheese and crispy ham topping:

3 wafer-thin slices Parma ham, all visible fat removed

2 tbsp grated reduced-fat Cheddar cheese

a handful of chives, snipped

freshly ground black pepper

1 Preheat the oven to 200°C, 400°F, gas mark 6.

2 Prick the potatoes all over with a fork. Put them in a baking pan, then lightly spray with oil and sprinkle with sea salt crystals. Bake in the preheated oven for 25–30 minutes until golden brown and crisp outside and soft inside. Remove and set aside until cool enough to handle.

3 Put the slices of Parma ham on a non-stick baking tray (cookie sheet) and cook in the preheated oven for about 5 minutes until crisp and golden. Alternatively, dry-fry in a non-stick frying pan (skillet).

4 Preheat the overhead grill (broiler). Split the potatoes in half lengthways and scoop out the insides. Mash with a fork and mix in the grated cheese and chives. Crumble in the Parma ham. Divide between the potato skins.

5 Pop the loaded potato skins under the hot grill for 3–4 minutes until the cheese melts.

Variation

CHEESY TOMATO TOPPING

And here's a veggie pizza-style variation.
You can make the sauce in advance.

....

SERVES 2

Prep: 5 minutes

Cook: 30–35 minutes

Per serving:

100 kcals

418 kJ

1.5g fat

High GI

low-cal spray oil

2 spring onions (scallions), chopped

2 garlic cloves, crushed

1 x 200g/7oz (scant 1 cup) can chopped tomatoes

sea salt and freshly ground black pepper

a few drops of balsamic vinegar

2 tbsp grated reduced-fat Cheddar cheese

a few basil leaves, torn

1 Lightly spray a saucepan with oil and cook the spring onions and garlic over a low to medium heat for 3–4 minutes until tender. Add the tomatoes and turn up the heat. Cook for at least 5 minutes until thickened and reduced. Season to taste with salt and pepper and a few drops of balsamic vinegar.

2 Preheat the overhead grill (broiler). Split the potatoes in half lengthways and scoop out the insides. Mash with a fork and stir into the tomato sauce. Pile the mixture into the potato skins and sprinkle with the grated cheese.

3 Place under the hot grill for 3–4 minutes until the cheese melts. Serve strewn with basil leaves.

CHILLI BAKED SWEET POTATOES

This spicy vegetarian chilli complements the natural sweetness of the sweet potatoes. You can use the chilli mixture to top two 175g/6oz jacket-baked regular potatoes – the calories will stay the same. The kidney beans add colour but you can substitute any canned beans – apart from baked beans, of course!

SERVES 2

Prep: 10 minutes

Cook: 45–50 mins

Per serving:

340 kcals

1423 kJ

3.7g fat

Low GI

2 x 150g/5oz sweet potatoes

low-cal spray oil

1 small onion, chopped

2 garlic cloves, crushed

1 small red (bell) pepper, deseeded and diced

2 tsp chilli powder

1 x 200g/7oz can (scant 1 cup) chopped tomatoes

1 x 200g/7oz can (generous 1 cup) red kidney beans, rinsed and drained

a few sprigs of parsley, chopped

sea salt and freshly ground black pepper

2 tbsp grated reduced-fat Cheddar cheese

1 Preheat the oven to 190°C, 375°F, gas mark 5.

2 Scrub the sweet potatoes and place them on a baking tray (cookie sheet). Bake in the preheated oven for 45–50 minutes until they feel tender when pressed gently.

3 Meanwhile, make the chilli. Lightly spray a saucepan with oil and set over a low heat. Add the onion, garlic and red pepper and cook gently, stirring occasionally, for about 8–10 minutes until tender.

4 Stir in the chilli powder and cook for 1 minute, then add the tomatoes and kidney beans. Simmer gently for 10–15 minutes until the mixture thickens and reduces. Stir in the parsley and season to taste with salt and pepper.

5 Split the potatoes in half or cut a cross in the top of each one and press gently on the sides to open it up. Spoon the chilli over the top and sprinkle with grated cheese.

FRUITY QUINOA SALAD *with* ROASTED VEGETABLES

Quinoa has become very popular in recent years due to its reputation as a 'super food'. It's gluten-free and a good source of protein and fibre, making it a great healthy food for slimmers. It has an interesting texture but rather a bland flavour so you might like to cook it in low-fat vegetable stock rather than water – the additional calories are negligible. This tastes even better if you scatter some coarsely chopped toasted cashews over the top, although each nut has 10 kcals and 1g fat!

SERVES 2

Prep: 15 minutes

Cook: 20–25 mins

Per serving:

310 kcals

1297 kJ

10g fat

Low GI

---

2 carrots, peeled and thickly sliced

1 small red onion, peeled and cut into wedges

low-cal spray oil

sea salt and freshly ground black pepper

60g/2oz (scant ½ cup) quinoa (dry weight)

2 tbsp light soy sauce

juice of 1 lime

a handful of coriander (cilantro), chopped

1 small mango, peeled, stoned (pitted) and chopped

1 baby avocado, peeled, stoned (pitted) and diced

seeds of ½ pomegranate

1 Preheat the oven to 190°C, 375°F, gas mark 5.

2 Arrange the carrots and red onion wedges in a roasting pan. Lightly spray with oil and season with salt and pepper. Roast in the preheated oven, turning occasionally, for 20–25 minutes until tender.

3 Meanwhile, cook the quinoa according to the instructions on the packet. Leave it to steam in the pan, off the heat, for a few minutes before fluffing up with a fork.

4 Stir the soy sauce and lime juice into the quinoa and then add the coriander, mango and avocado. Check the seasoning.

5 Divide between 2 shallow serving dishes and top with the roasted vegetables. Scatter the pomegranate seeds over the top and serve warm.

CHEAT'S QUICK 'N' EASY PIZZAS

SERVES 2

Prep: 10 minutes

Cook: 20 minutes

Even a single slice of a take-out pizza can be as much as 400–500 kcals, so it's much healthier to make your own. You don't need special pizza bases to make these delicious mini pizzas – just use English muffins instead. Or you can toast 2 mini pitta breads per person and the calories will stay approximately the same.

Per serving:

245 kcals

1025 kJ

6.7g fat

Medium GI

low-cal spray oil

2 garlic cloves, crushed

½ red onion, finely diced

2 tsp tomato paste

1 x 200g/7oz can (1 generous cup) chopped tomatoes

a few basil leaves, chopped

sea salt and freshly ground black pepper

a few drops of balsamic vinegar (optional)

2 x 57g/2oz English muffins

60g/2oz reduced-fat mozzarella cheese, thinly sliced

4 black olives, stoned (pitted)

1 Lightly spray a frying pan (skillet) with oil and set over a low to medium heat. Cook the garlic and onion for 6–8 minutes until the onion is softened.

2 Stir in the tomato paste, tomatoes and basil, and cook for about 10 minutes until the mixture thickens and reduces. Season to taste with salt and pepper and add a few drops of balsamic vinegar (if using) to add sweetness.

3 Split the muffins in half and lightly toast them. Spread the tomato mixture over them right up to the edges and cover with the mozzarella slices. Top each pizza with an olive.

4 Place under a really hot grill (broiler) for 3–4 minutes until the cheese melts and is turning slightly golden.

5 Grind a little black pepper over the top and serve immediately, with a salad.

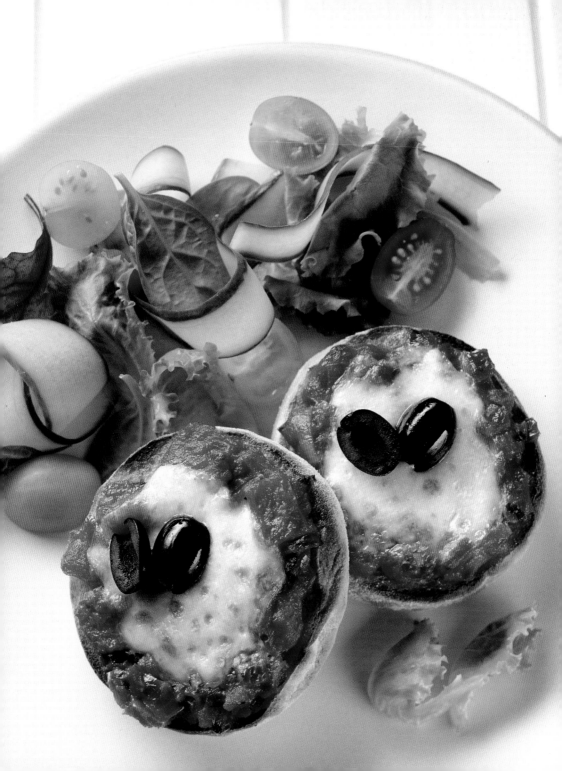

CHEAT'S BEANS *on* TOAST

SERVES 2

Prep: 5 minutes

Cook: 10–13 mins

Per serving:

175 kcals

732 kJ

1.3g fat

Medium GI

This may take longer than opening a can and warming up the contents but it really is easy and it's ready in 15 minutes. If you don't have any butterbeans (lima beans) in the cupboard, don't worry. Any canned beans will work well and the calories will stay roughly the same. Add another slice of toast and the kcals will be 230 per serving. Enjoy!

low-cal spray oil

1 small red onion, finely chopped

1 garlic clove, crushed

100g/3½oz fresh cherry or baby plum tomatoes, diced

1 tsp tomato paste

1 x 200g/7oz can (3 cups) butterbeans (lima beans), rinsed and drained

a dash of balsamic vinegar

sea salt and freshly ground black pepper

2 x 25g/1oz slices wholemeal bread

2 tbsp finely chopped parsley or basil

1 Lightly spray a pan with oil and set over a low to medium heat. Add the red onion and garlic and cook for 6–8 minutes, stirring occasionally, until really tender and golden.

2 Add the tomatoes and cook for 2–3 minutes over a medium heat. Stir in the tomato paste and butterbeans and warm through gently. Add a few drops of balsamic vinegar to taste and some salt and pepper.

3 Lightly toast the bread and spoon the beans over the top. Sprinkle with herbs and serve immediately.

TIP: You can spice this up by adding a diced chilli when you're cooking the onion and garlic.

CHEAT'S TUNA MELT 'TOASTIES'

SERVES 2

Prep: 10 minutes

Cook: 5 minutes

Per serving:

245 kcals

1025 kJ

6.7g fat

Medium GI

A tuna melt from a café or coffee shop usually works out at around 400–500 kcals! Our low-calorie version tastes just as good, if not better. Always use canned tuna in spring water – not oil – and extra light (or lighter than light) mayo (the calories will be about one-third of light mayonnaise).

1 x 160g/5oz can tuna in spring water, drained

4 spring onions (scallions), chopped

2 tbsp extra light mayonnaise

freshly ground black pepper

2 x 30g/1oz slices multigrain bread

60g/2oz reduced-fat Cheddar cheese, grated

1 Preheat an overhead grill (broiler). Mash the tuna and stir in the spring onions and mayo. Season with plenty of ground black pepper.

2 Lightly toast the bread and spread the tuna mayo mixture over one side of each slice, right up to the edges.

3 Sprinkle the grated cheese over the top and pop under the really hot grill for 3–4 minutes until the cheese is bubbling and golden brown.

4 Cut each toastie into halves or quarters and eat immediately.

CHEAT'S CRISPY CHICKEN NUGGETS

These crisp cheesy chicken nuggets are delicious and much healthier and lower in fat than take-out or frozen ones. You can cook them in a hot pan, lightly sprayed with oil, over a medium heat if preferred. Cheat's butternut squash 'fries' make a great low-fat accompaniment (see page 108).

SERVES 2

Prep: 15 minutes

Chill: 15 minutes

Cook: 15 minutes

Per serving:

270 kcals

1130 kJ

6g fat

Medium GI

250g/9oz skinned, boned chicken breasts, cut into large chunks

1 tsp flour

1 small free-range egg, beaten

40g/1½oz (scant 1 cup) fresh white breadcrumbs

2 tbsp grated Parmesan cheese

a good pinch of cayenne pepper

low-cal spray oil

sea salt crystals and freshly ground black pepper

2 tbsp tomato ketchup

1 Preheat the oven to 200°C, 400°F, gas mark 6. Dust the chicken lightly with flour and then dip into the beaten egg.

2 Mix the breadcrumbs, grated Parmesan and cayenne in a shallow dish and add the chicken, turning it until coated all over with the mixture.

3 Place the coated chicken on a plate, cover with cling film (plastic wrap) and chill in the fridge for at least 15 minutes.

4 Arrange the chicken on a non-stick baking tray (cookie sheet) and lightly spray with oil. Bake in the preheated oven for about 15 minutes, turning once, until golden brown and crisp on the outside and cooked right through.

5 Sprinkle with sea salt and black pepper, and serve immediately with the tomato ketchup and some steamed green vegetables or a salad.

CHEAT'S CHICKEN CAESAR SALAD

The average Caesar salad is very high in calories as the dressing is made with olive oil and the croutons are fried in butter or oil. Our cheat's version is not only healthy and low in fat but also delicious – you can enjoy it without worrying about your waistline. If you like anchovies in your Caesar salad, drain off the oil and rinse them before using. Each anchovy will add 8 kcals and 0.5g fat.

SERVES 2

Prep: 15 minutes

Cook: 6–8 minutes

Per serving:

290 kcals

1213 kJ

6.5g fat

Medium GI

2 x 30g/1oz slices stale bread

low-cal spray oil

200g/7oz skinned chicken breast fillets

1 head cos (Romaine) lettuce, roughly shredded

2 tbsp grated Parmesan cheese

For the Caesar dressing:

3 tbsp oil-free vinaigrette (see page 53)

grated zest and juice of 1 lemon

1 large garlic clove, crushed

a few drops of Worcestershire sauce

1 small free-range egg yolk

sea salt and freshly ground black pepper

1 Preheat the oven to 150°C, 300°F, gas mark 2.

2 Cut the bread into small cubes or tear into pieces. Place on a baking tray (cookie sheet) and lightly spray with oil. Bake in the preheated oven for about 10 minutes until the croutons are golden and crisp.

3 Meanwhile, lightly spray a ridged griddle pan with oil and set over a medium heat. When the pan is hot, add the chicken and cook, turning occasionally, for about 8–10 minutes until cooked right through, golden brown and attractively striped.

4 Make the Caesar dressing: mix together the vinaigrette, lemon zest and juice, garlic and Worcestershire sauce. Beat in the egg yolk and season with salt and pepper.

5 Toss the lettuce and croutons in the dressing and divide the salad between 2 serving plates.

6 Cut the chicken into thin slices or cubes and scatter over the top. Sprinkle with the Parmesan and serve.

CHEAT'S HAMBURGERS

SERVES 2

Prep: 10 minutes

Cook: 8–10 mins

Per serving:

310 kcals

1297 kJ

8.3g fat

High GI

Do make sure you use only extra-lean minced (ground) beef with minimal fat. It will have half the fat and 50 fewer kcals than lean mince, and a whopping 13g fat and 120 kcals less than regular minced beef. Serve each burger with 1 tablespoon of tomato ketchup and you'll add 18 kcals per serving. If you love cheeseburgers and add a single 15g/½oz slice of Edam or Swiss cheese to each burger, you'll have about 40–50 extra kcals and 3–4g fat. If using burger buns, check the labels carefully: most have around 160 kcals (50 kcals more than the wholemeal rolls we've used).

225g/8oz (1 cup) extra-lean minced (ground) beef (less than 5% fat)

1 small onion, grated

1 tbsp tomato ketchup

a few drops of Worcestershire sauce

1 small egg, beaten

sea salt and freshly ground black pepper

low-cal spray oil

2 x 45g/1½oz wholemeal rolls

a few crisp lettuce leaves

1 ripe tomato, thinly sliced

2 pickled gherkins (dill pickles), sliced

1 Preheat an overhead grill (broiler) or light the barbecue.

2 Mix the minced beef, onion, tomato ketchup, Worcestershire sauce and most of the beaten egg in a bowl. Season with salt and pepper.

3 Divide the mixture into 2 equal portions and shape each one with your hands into a thick burger. Spray lightly with oil.

4 Place the burgers on a rack under the hot grill (broiler) or on the preheated hot barbecue and cook for about 4–5 minutes each side, depending on how well you like them cooked. They should be well coloured and slightly charred on the outside but juicy and moist inside.

5 Split the rolls and fill with the lettuce, sliced tomato, gherkins and burgers. Serve with a salad.

CHEAT'S STEAK 'SANDWICH'

SERVES 2

Prep: 10 minutes

Cook: 10 minutes

Per serving:

240 kcals

1004 kJ

4.8g fat

Low GI

We've sandwiched our steak between grilled (broiled) mushrooms instead of bread. Large portobello mushrooms are surprisingly 'meaty' and filling. Each large cap has 32 kcals compared to 100 in an average slice of white bread. If wished, you can serve the 'sandwiches' with mustard – a teaspoon averages 8 kcals and 0.5g fat.

2 x 100g/3½oz lean fillet (filet mignon) or sirloin steaks, all visible fat removed

sea salt and freshly ground black pepper

4 large portobello (or field) mushrooms

low-cal spray oil

2 garlic cloves, crushed

For the 'cheat's pesto':

4 tbsp 0% fat Greek yoghurt

a few sprigs of basil, finely chopped

4 ripe cherry tomatoes, skinned and diced

1 Season the steaks with salt and pepper and cook under a preheated hot grill (broiler) or in a griddle pan lightly sprayed with oil and set over a medium to high heat for about 3–5 minutes each side, depending on whether you like your steak rare or well done.

2 Meanwhile, remove the stalks from the portobello mushroom caps and spray each mushroom lightly with oil. Grill (broil) until golden brown and softened underneath and then turn the mushrooms over, fill each one with a crushed garlic clove and grind over some salt and pepper. Grill for about 5 minutes until cooked and tender.

3 In a bowl, mix together all the ingredients for the pesto.

4 Take 2 serving plates and place a cooked mushroom (garlic side up) on each one. Put a little pesto in the hollow in the centre and place a steak on top. Spread with the remaining pesto, then cover with the other mushroom cap to create a 'sandwich'. Serve immediately, with a green salad.

CHEAT'S CRUNCHY FISH FINGERS

SERVES 2

Prep: 15 minutes

Cook: 8–10 mins

Per serving:

225 kcals

941 kJ

3g fat

Medium GI

These homemade low-fat fish fingers look and taste fabulous and are surprisingly filling. One portion has approximately 100 fewer kcals than bought commercial ones. Instead of grilling (broiling) them, you can bake them in an oven preheated to 190°C, 375°F, gas mark 5 – whichever you prefer. Serve them with extra light mayonnaise instead of ketchup and you'll add approximately 1–2g fat per serving, but the calories will stay roughly the same.

300g/10oz white fish fillets, e.g. cod
or haddock, pin-boned and skinned

1 tsp flour for dusting

1 medium free-range egg white

45g/1½oz (scant 1 cup) fresh white breadcrumbs

sea salt and freshly ground black pepper

low-cal spray oil

2 tbsp tomato ketchup

1 Cut the fish fillets into thick strips and dust them lightly with flour.

2 In a clean, dry bowl, beat the egg white until stiff. Dip the strips of fish into the beaten egg white.

3 Spread out the breadcrumbs in a large, shallow dish and coat the fish fingers in them. Season with salt and pepper, arrange them in a foil-lined grill (broiler) pan and lightly spray with oil.

4 Cook under a preheated hot grill (broiler) for 4–5 minutes each side, until the fish fingers are golden brown and crisp on the outside but thoroughly cooked on the inside.

5 Serve the fish fingers with the tomato ketchup, and a green vegetable of your choice.

CHEESY CHICKEN QUESADILLAS

Quesadillas are surprisingly filling and so easy and quick to make. You can use cold leftover roast chicken or buy a ready-cooked breast from the supermarket. If you don't want to go to the trouble of roasting the red (bell) pepper, just use the bottled flamed ones – drain and dice. Check the labels carefully when buying tortilla wraps; you are looking for 120 kcals max per tortilla. Some can be as high as 200!

SERVES 2

Prep: 15 minutes

Cook: 4–6 minutes

Per serving:

350 kcals

1464 kJ

10g fat

Medium GI

150g/5oz cooked chicken breast, skinned and diced

1 roasted red (bell) pepper, deseeded and diced

2 spring onions (scallions), finely chopped

1 small red chilli, deseeded and diced

a few sprigs of coriander (cilantro), finely chopped

sea salt and freshly ground black pepper

2 x 40g/1½oz soft flour tortillas

60g/2oz (generous ½ cup) reduced-fat Cheddar cheese, grated

low-cal spray oil

4 tbsp fresh salsa

2 tbsp 0% fat Greek yoghurt

2 tbsp reduced-fat guacamole

1 In a bowl mix together the chicken, red pepper, spring onions, chilli and coriander. Season lightly with salt and pepper.

2 Divide the mixture between the tortillas and sprinkle the grated cheese over the top. Fold each tortilla over into a half-moon shape to enclose the filling and press firmly around the edges.

3 Lightly spray a heavy griddle pan with oil and set over a medium heat. When it's hot, place the tortillas in the pan and cook for 2–3 minutes each side until they are warmed through, golden and slightly crisp and the cheese has melted and is starting to ooze.

4 Serve the quesadillas cut into wedges with the salsa, yoghurt and guacamole.

Variation

REFRIED BEAN QUESADILLAS

Here's a delicious veggie alternative to the chicken recipe opposite.

....

SERVES 2

Prep: 10 minutes

Cook: 10–12 mins

Per serving:

350 kcals

1464 kJ

9.7g fat

Medium GI

low-cal spray oil

4 spring onions (scallions), finely chopped

2 garlic cloves, crushed

½ tsp cumin seeds

a pinch of chilli powder

200g/7oz (generous 3 cups) red kidney beans, rinsed and drained

2 x 40g/1½oz soft flour tortillas

a handful of coriander (cilantro), chopped

sea salt and freshly ground black pepper

60g/2oz (½ cup) grated reduced-fat Cheddar cheese

4 tbsp fresh salsa

2 tbsp 0% fat Greek yoghurt

2 tbsp reduced-fat guacamole

1 Lightly spray a frying pan (skillet) with oil and set over a medium heat. Cook the spring onions and garlic for 2 minutes. Stir in the cumin seeds, chilli powder and beans and warm through gently for 4–5 minutes. Mash everything coarsely with a potato masher and stir in the coriander. Season to taste.

2 Divide the mixture between the tortillas and sprinkle with the cheese. Top with the salsa and then fold each tortilla over into a half-moon shape to enclose the filling, and press firmly around the edges.

3 Cook as opposite and serve hot, cut into wedges, with the yoghurt and guacamole.

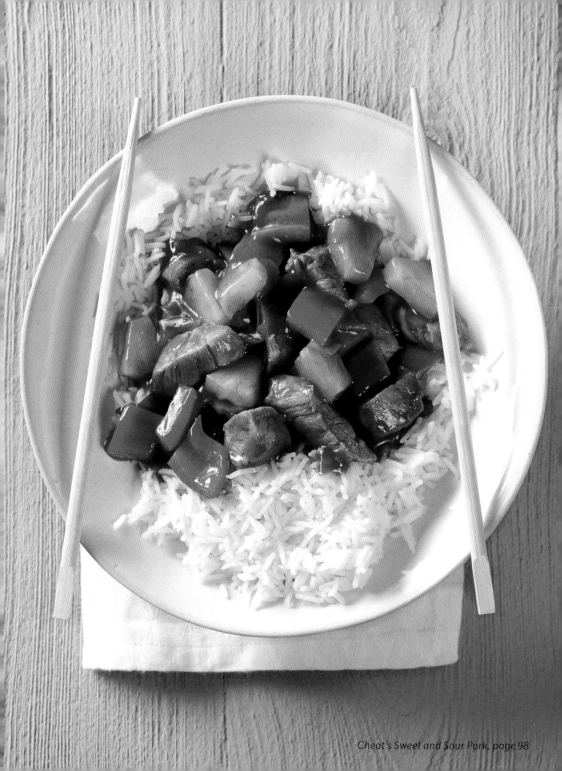

Cheat's Sweet and Sour Pork, page 98

Meals in minutes

(main meals & suppers)

GREEN RECIPES (MAX 400 KCALS)

Chicken shawarma with cheat's aubergine fries

Chicken cacciatore with smashed butterbeans

Chicken and spinach towers

Turkey and clementine stir-fry

Thai green curried chicken tray bake

Grilled fish with Puy lentils

Lemon chicken souvlaki with greens

Cheat's lentil and vegetable cottage pie

Spiced dhal with roasted vegetables

Cheat's 'rice' with Mexican griddled prawns

Cheat's chicken lasagne

Cheat's chicken tikka masala

Cheat's 'pasta' with soy and garlic chicken drumsticks

Cheat's tandoori chicken with chana dhal

Cheat's fish and chips

AMBER RECIPES (MAX 450 KCALS)

Chicken pasta bake

Chicken saltimbocca with lemony smashed pesto potatoes

Thai green prawn and coconut curry

Shrimp scampi

Crispy baked salmon and spinach

Japanese griddled tuna steaks and brown rice

Cheat's sweet and sour pork

Spicy stir-fried quinoa

Cheat's spaghetti bolognese

Cheat's chilli con carne

Cheat's pad Thai

Cheat's seafood risotto

Cheat's macaroni cheese

Skinny lasagne stacks

CHICKEN SHAWARMA *with* CHEAT'S AUBERGINE FRIES

Spicy, aromatic chicken shawarma is popular as a snack or main dish throughout the Levant. It's usually served in pitta bread with pickled cucumber, pungent garlic sauce and salad, but we've created our own delicious slimming version with cheat's aubergine (eggplant) 'fries' and fennel yoghurt. You can use the feathery fronds on top of a fennel bulb to flavour the yoghurt and even add some diced fennel. If you don't have any fennel, try dill instead.

SERVES 2

Prep: 15 minutes

Chill: 1 hour minimum

Cook: 30–40 minutes

Per serving:

300 kcals

1255 kJ

3g fat

Low GI

2 x 150g/5oz skinned, boned chicken breasts

1 x 300g/10oz aubergine (eggplant)

low-cal spray oil

a pinch of cayenne pepper

sea salt and freshly ground black pepper

1 tsp fennel seeds

120g/4oz (½ cup) 0% fat Greek yoghurt

a few sprigs of fennel herb, finely chopped

a squeeze of lemon juice

2 sprigs of cherry tomatoes on the vine

For the shawarma marinade:

4 tbsp 0% fat Greek yoghurt

juice of 1 lemon

3 garlic cloves, crushed

1 tsp grated fresh root ginger

1 tsp ground cumin

1 tsp paprika

a pinch of ground nutmeg

¼ tsp dried oregano or thyme

a good pinch of salt

1 Mix together all the ingredients for the shawarma marinade in a shallow dish.

2 Cut each chicken breast in half horizontally so you have 2 thin escalopes (or bash each with a rolling pin between 2 sheets of baking parchment to flatten it out). Add to the marinade and coat the chicken all over. Cover the dish and leave in the fridge for at least 1 hour (overnight, if wished).

3 Preheat the oven to 200°C, 400°F, gas 6 and make the aubergine fries: cut the aubergine in half lengthways and then cut each half into long matchsticks. Arrange them on a non-stick baking tray (cookie sheet) and lightly spray with oil. Sprinkle with cayenne and a little sea salt. Bake in the preheated oven for 30–40 minutes until crisp and golden brown.

4 Meanwhile, heat a small frying pan (skillet) over a high heat. Add the fennel seeds and cook for about 1 minute, tossing them occasionally, until golden brown and they release their aroma. Remove from the pan immediately before they burn and stir into the yoghurt with the chopped fennel herb and lemon juice. Season with salt and pepper.

5 Set a griddle pan over a high heat and, when it's really hot, add the marinated chicken. Cook for 4–5 minutes each side until golden brown and thoroughly cooked inside. Remove from the pan and griddle the tomatoes until they are starting to soften and char.

6 Cut the chicken into really thin slices and serve immediately with the griddled tomatoes, aubergine fries and fennel yoghurt.

Amber option: Divide the chicken between 2 split warmed, griddled 60g/2oz wholemeal pitta breads. This will add approximately 140 kcals and 1g fat per serving.

CHICKEN CACCIATORE *with* SMASHED BUTTERBEANS

This 'hunter's' chicken stew is enjoyed all over Italy. The smashed beans soak up the sauce and are a nutritious alternative to potatoes or rice. Try adding some baby spinach leaves for an attractively green-flecked variation. Just stir a handful into the cooked onion with the blitzed bean purée and heat through as directed below.

SERVES 2

Prep: 15 minutes

Cook: 15 minutes

Per serving:

400 kcals

1674 kJ

3.5g fat

Low GI

---

2 x 125g/4oz skinned, boned chicken breasts

1 tsp flour

low-cal spray oil

4 garlic cloves, crushed

2 carrots, diced

a few sprigs of rosemary, plus extra to garnish

360ml/12fl oz (1½ cups) chicken stock

200g/7oz juicy tomatoes, chopped

sea salt and freshly ground black pepper

For the smashed beans:

low-cal spray oil

1 small onion, diced

a sprig of rosemary

1 x 400g/14oz can (generous 5 cups) butterbeans (lima beans), rinsed and drained

grated zest of 1 lemon

1 Lightly dust the chicken with the flour. Lightly spray a deep frying pan (skillet) with oil and set over a medium heat. Add the chicken to the hot pan and cook, turning occasionally, for 4–5 minutes until golden brown on both sides. Remove and keep warm.

2 Add the garlic and carrots and cook for 2–3 minutes. Return the chicken to the pan and add the rosemary, stock and tomatoes. Cover with a lid and simmer gently for 40–45 minutes until the chicken is cooked through and the sauce has reduced. Season with salt and pepper.

3 Meanwhile, make the smashed beans: lightly spray a small pan with oil and gently cook the onion and rosemary over a low heat, stirring occasionally, for about 10 minutes until really tender. Remove the rosemary sprigs and blitz the leaves with the beans and lemon zest in a blender or food processor until you have a thick, coarse-textured purée.

4 Add the purée to the onion in the pan, stir well and heat through gently for a few minutes. Season to taste with salt and pepper.

5 Divide the chicken and sauce between 2 serving plates. Serve garnished with rosemary, with the smashed beans.

TIP: You can use canned cannellini beans instead of butterbeans.

CHICKEN *and* SPINACH TOWERS

You could substitute two 100g/3½oz really lean sirloin steaks (all visible fat removed) for the chicken breasts. Cook in the same way and the calories will stay the same (you'll have 6g fat per serving).

SERVES 2

Prep: 10 minutes

Cook: 25 minutes

Per serving:

400 kcals

1674 kJ

4.5g fat

High GI

400g/14oz baby spinach leaves

1 tbsp water

a good pinch of grated nutmeg

4 tbsp 0% fat Greek yoghurt

low-cal spray oil

2 x 125g/4oz chicken breasts, skinned and boned

sea salt and freshly ground black pepper

2 baked jacket potatoes (125g/4oz each uncooked weight), to serve

snipped chives, to garnish

For the red onion and balsamic marmalade:

low-cal spray oil

1 red onion, thinly sliced

1 tsp soft brown sugar

2 tsp balsamic vinegar

1 Make the red onion and balsamic marmalade: lightly spray a non-stick frying pan (skillet) with oil and set over a low heat. Add the onion to the hot pan and cook very gently for about 15 minutes, stirring occasionally, until it's really tender and starting to caramelise. Stir in the remaining ingredients and cook gently for 10 minutes. Season lightly with salt and pepper.

2 Put the spinach in a large saucepan with the water. Set over a low to medium heat and cover with a lid. Cook for 2–3 minutes, shaking the pan occasionally, until the leaves wilt and turn bright green. Remove from the heat immediately and drain in a colander, pressing down with a saucer to squeeze out all the moisture. Return to the warm pan and stir in the nutmeg and half the yoghurt. Season to taste and keep warm.

3 Lightly spray a frying pan or ridged griddle pan with oil and set over a medium heat. Cook the chicken breasts for about 15 minutes, turning them halfway through, until golden brown and thoroughly cooked.

4 Arrange the spinach neatly on each serving plate and cover with a chicken breast. Top with a spoonful of red onion marmalade. Serve with the baked potatoes, topped with the remaining yoghurt and chives.

TURKEY *and* CLEMENTINE STIR-FRY

You can use turkey or chicken breast meat in this fruity stir-fry. It's very refreshing on cold winter days, especially at Christmas, when you're tired of eating rich, stodgy food and fancy something lighter. Even though there are no carbs, this will leave you feeling satisfied and full.

SERVES 2

Prep: 10 minutes

Cook: 10 minutes

Per serving:

320 kcals

1339 kJ

4.8g fat

Low GI

low-cal spray oil

300g/10oz skinned turkey breast, thinly sliced

2 garlic cloves, crushed

1 red chilli, deseeded and diced

300g/10oz white mushrooms, sliced

1 red (bell) pepper, deseeded and sliced

4 spring onions (scallions), sliced

200g/7oz (2 cups) bean sprouts

200g/7oz pak choi (bok choy), coarsely sliced

a few sprigs of coriander (cilantro), chopped (optional)

For the clementine and ginger dressing:

2 tbsp soy sauce

grated zest and juice of 2 clementines

peeled segments of 2 clementines

2 tsp grated fresh root ginger

sea salt and freshly ground black pepper

1 Lightly spray a wok or deep frying pan (skillet) with oil and set over a medium to high heat. Add the turkey and stir-fry briskly for 4–5 minutes until golden brown all over.

2 Add the garlic and chilli and stir-fry for 1 minute. Next add the mushrooms, red pepper, spring onions, bean sprouts and pak choi. Stir-fry for 3–4 minutes until the vegetables are just tender but still crisp and the turkey is cooked right through.

3 Mix all the ingredients together for the clementine and ginger dressing in a bowl, adding salt and pepper to taste. Add to the turkey and vegetables and heat through gently.

4 Divide the stir-fry between 2 shallow serving bowls and serve immediately.

Amber option: Serve this stir-fry with 60g/2oz egg noodles (dry weight) and you'll add 105 kcals and 0.6g fat per serving. Just cook the noodles according to the packet instructions and stir into the wok with the dressing.

> TIP: You can use satsumas or mandarins instead of clementines.

THAI GREEN CURRIED CHICKEN TRAY BAKE

The great thing about this supper is that it's all cooked in the same pan, so there's hardly any washing up. It's worth making the curry paste yourself as the flavour is so much better and more aromatic than shop-bought versions. And it's fat-free.

SERVES 2

Prep: 15 minutes

Cook: 35 minutes

Per serving:

400 kcals

1674 kJ

10.8g fat

Medium GI

4 x 90g/3oz chicken thighs, skinned and boned

1 red onion, peeled and quartered

1 red (bell) pepper, deseeded and cut into chunks

1 yellow (bell) pepper, deseeded and cut into chunks

200g/7oz sweet potato, peeled and cut into wedges

low-cal spray oil

freshly ground black pepper

a small handful of coriander (cilantro), chopped

For the Thai green curry paste:

2.5cm/1in fresh root ginger, peeled and chopped

2 garlic cloves, peeled

2 lemongrass stalks, peeled and chopped

1 red chilli, diced

grated zest and juice of 1 lime

2 tsp nam pla (Thai fish sauce)

1 small bunch of coriander (cilantro), chopped

1 Preheat the oven to 200°C, 400°F, gas mark 6.

2 Put all the ingredients for the Thai green curry paste in a blender and blitz until you have a smooth paste. Rub this into the chicken thighs.

3 Arrange the chicken, red onion, peppers and sweet potato in an ovenproof dish or roasting pan. Lightly spray with oil and grind some black pepper over the top. Bake in the preheated oven, turning the chicken and vegetables once or twice, for about 35 minutes or until the chicken is cooked right through and the vegetables are tender.

4 Divide between 2 serving plates and serve immediately, sprinkled with chopped coriander.

GRILLED FISH
with PUY LENTILS

If you can't find Puy lentils, use the brown or green sort instead – the small red ones won't work as they lose their shape as they cook. Any skinned and boned white fish fillets are suitable, including monkfish (angler fish) or sea bass. The calories will stay roughly the same.

SERVES 2

Prep: 10 minutes

Cook: 25 minutes

Per serving:

350 kcals

1464 kJ

4.2g fat

Low GI

100g/3½oz (½ cup) Puy lentils

1 carrot, diced

2 celery sticks, diced

4 spring onions (scallions), thinly sliced

a handful of parsley, chopped

juice of 1 lemon

a few drops of balsamic vinegar

sea salt and freshly ground black pepper

2 x 150g/5oz cod or haddock fillets, pin-boned and skinned

200g/7oz courgettes (zucchini)

1 Rinse the lentils in a sieve under cold running water. Put them in a saucepan with the carrot, celery and enough cold water to cover them. Bring to the boil, then reduce the heat and simmer gently, covered, for 15–20 minutes or until the lentils and vegetables are cooked and tender but not mushy. The lentils should keep their shape and have a little 'bite'.

2 Drain well and stir the spring onions, parsley and lemon juice into the lentil and vegetable mixture. Add a few drops of balsamic vinegar and season to taste with salt and pepper.

3 Meanwhile, cook the fish fillets under a preheated overhead grill (broiler) for 3–4 minutes each side until cooked right through. Alternatively, wrap them in foil and cook in a moderate oven (180°C, 350°F, gas mark 4) for 15 minutes.

4 Using a potato peeler, thinly slice the courgettes lengthways into long, thin ribbons. Cook in a pan of boiling water or steam them for 2 minutes until just tender but not too soft – you want them to keep their shape and fresh colour.

5 Divide the warm lentil mixture between 2 serving plates and place the fish on top. Serve immediately with the courgette ribbons.

LEMON CHICKEN SOUVLAKI *with* GREENS

This traditional Greek dish is simple to make, tastes great and is so healthy and slimming, too. The spring greens, known as horta in Greece, are sometimes served at room temperature or cold. You can use spinach, wild dandelion leaves or any edible green leaves.

SERVES 2

Prep: 10 minutes

Chill: 15 minutes

Cook: 10 minutes

Per serving:

340 kcals

1423 kJ

6g fat

Low GI

1 tsp fennel seeds

a good pinch of dried oregano or thyme

grated zest and juice of 1 lemon

400g/14oz chicken breast fillets, cut into chunks

4 thick woody sprigs of rosemary, most of the leaves removed (optional)

low-cal spray oil

2 courgettes (zucchini), sliced diagonally

a handful of parsley, chopped

4 tbsp low-fat tzatziki

For the greens:

low-cal spray oil

2 garlic cloves, crushed

a pinch of dried chilli flakes (optional)

200g/7oz spring greens, shredded

1 small bunch of dill or flat-leaf parsley, chopped

juice of 1 small lemon

sea salt and freshly ground black pepper

1 Crush the fennel seeds with a pestle and mortar, tip into a bowl and stir in the dried herbs, lemon zest and juice. Add the chicken and stir into the lemony mixture.

2 Thread the chicken onto 4 sprigs of rosemary (or use wooden skewers that have been soaked in water for about 30 minutes to prevent them burning). Cover and chill in the fridge for 15 minutes.

3 Lightly spray the chicken skewers with oil and cook under a preheated hot grill (broiler) or over hot coals on a barbecue for about 10 minutes, turning occasionally, until golden brown and thoroughly cooked right through.

4 Meanwhile, for the greens, lightly spray a wok or deep frying pan (skillet) with oil and set over a high heat. Add the garlic and chilli flakes (if using) and cook for 1 minute. Add the spring greens and stir-fry for 2–3 minutes until just tender (they should retain a little 'bite'). Stir in the herbs and lemon juice and season to taste.

5 Cook the courgettes in a hot ridged griddle pan over a medium to high heat for 2–3 minutes until just tender and attractively striped.

6 Serve the chicken skewers sprinkled with chopped parsley, and with the tzatziki, courgettes and spring greens.

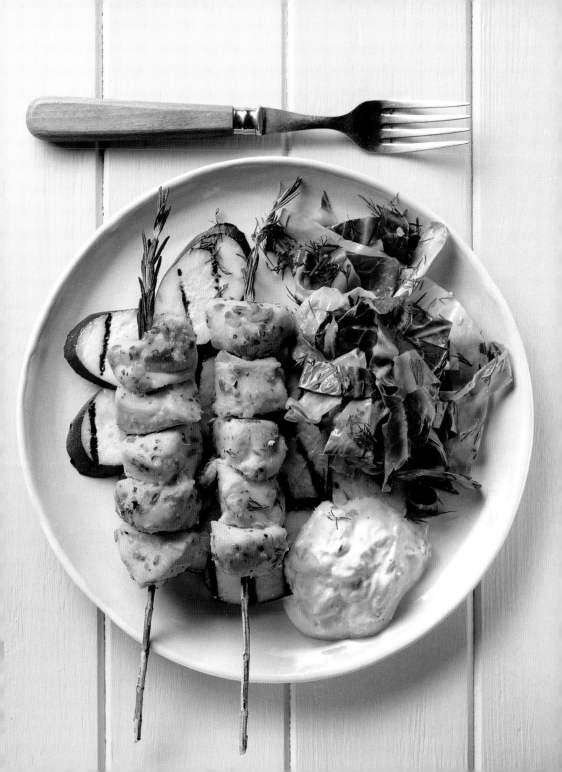

CHEAT'S LENTIL *and* VEGETABLE COTTAGE PIE

A really healthy veggie cottage pie topped with swede (rutabaga), which has a fraction of the calories of mashed potatoes. The reduced-fat Cheddar cheese adds the finishing touches of crispness and flavour but as it's actually an 'amber' food (see page 12) you may prefer to leave it out and save 15 kcals and 1g fat per serving.

SERVES 2

Prep: 15 minutes

Cook: 50–55 mins

Per serving:

400 kcals

1674 kJ

5g fat

Low GI

low-cal spray oil

1 leek, washed, trimmed and sliced

2 garlic cloves, crushed

2 carrots, diced

200g/7oz mushrooms, quartered

1 x 400g/14oz can (scant 2 cups) chopped tomatoes

120ml/4fl oz (½ cup) vegetable stock

1 x 400g/14oz can (scant 4 cups) green lentils, rinsed and drained

100g/3½oz baby spinach leaves

sea salt and freshly ground black pepper

a few drops of balsamic vinegar

For the topping:

400g/14oz swede (rutabaga), peeled and cubed

2 tbsp 0% fat Greek yoghurt

2 tbsp skimmed milk

1 tbsp grated reduced-fat Cheddar cheese

1 Preheat the oven to 200°C, 400°F, gas mark 6.

2 Lightly spray a saucepan with oil and set it over a low heat. Add the leek, garlic and carrots and cook, stirring occasionally, for about 10 minutes until tender. Add the mushrooms and cook for 5 minutes.

3 Add the tomatoes and stock and bring to the boil. Reduce the heat, stir in the lentils and simmer gently for 15 minutes until the sauce reduces and thickens and all the vegetables are cooked. Stir in the spinach and cook for 1 minute until it wilts. Season with salt and pepper and a few drops of balsamic vinegar.

4 Meanwhile, cook the swede in a pan of boiling water until tender. Drain well and mash coarsely with the yoghurt and milk. Season with salt and pepper.

5 Spoon the lentil and vegetable mixture into an ovenproof dish and cover with the mashed swede right up to the edges. Sprinkle with the Cheddar cheese and bake in the preheated oven for 20–25 minutes until bubbling and the top is crisp and golden brown. Serve immediately.

SPICED DHAL *with* ROASTED VEGETABLES

A bowl of steaming dhal is real comfort food and warming on a cold day. Lentils are surprisingly filling and a great source of protein, vitamins, minerals and dietary fibre. If you don't like the aniseed taste of fennel, you can use celeriac, aubergine (eggplant), courgettes (zucchini) or mushrooms instead. The calories will stay approximately the same.

SERVES 2

Prep: 15 minutes

Cook: 25–30 mins

Per serving:

390 kcals

1632 kJ

4.5g fat

Low GI

low-cal spray oil

1 small onion, sliced

2 garlic cloves, crushed

2 tsp grated fresh root ginger

1 red chilli, diced

1 tsp ground turmeric

1 tsp garam masala

150g/5oz (¾ cup) split red lentils (dry weight)

300ml/½ pint (1¼ cups) vegetable stock

2 ripe tomatoes, roughly chopped

juice of 1 lime

a handful of coriander (cilantro), chopped

For the roasted vegetables:

1 fennel bulb, cut into wedges

1 red onion, cut into wedges

2 carrots, cut into chunks

1 tsp cumin or coriander seeds

2 sprigs of rosemary

2 sprigs of sage

low-cal spray oil

sea salt and freshly ground black pepper

1 Preheat the oven to 200°C, 400°F, gas mark 6.

2 Put the fennel, red onion and carrots in a roasting pan and sprinkle with the seeds. Tuck the herbs down between the vegetables and spray lightly with oil. Season with salt and pepper and cook in the preheated oven for 25–30 minutes, turning them once or twice, until tender.

3 Meanwhile, lightly spray a saucepan with oil and cook the sliced onion, garlic, ginger and chilli over a medium heat for 4–5 minutes without colouring. Stir in the spices and cook for 1 minute.

4 Add the lentils and stock. Bring to the boil, then reduce the heat and simmer gently for 15 minutes, stirring occasionally.

5 Add the tomatoes and cook for 5–10 minutes or until the lentils break down and the dhal thickens – if it's too thick and the lentils are still hard, just add some more stock or water. Stir in the lime juice and chopped coriander, and season to taste with salt and pepper.

6 Divide the hot dhal between 2 shallow bowls and arrange the roasted vegetables on top. Serve immediately.

CHEAT'S 'RICE' *with* MEXICAN GRIDDLED PRAWNS

Beetroot (beet) 'rice' is low-fat and a fraction of the calories of real rice. It tastes delicious tossed in a fruity dressing. Some supermarkets even sell it in ready-prepared packs to save you blitzing the beetroot yourself.

SERVES 2

Prep: 25 minutes

Cook: 10–15 mins

Per serving:

380 kcals

1590 kJ

9g fat

Low GI

200g/7oz raw large prawns (jumbo shrimp)

juice of 1 lime

1 red chilli, deseeded and diced

2 tbsp chopped parsley, coriander (cilantro) or chives

freshly ground black pepper

low-cal spray oil

1 green (bell) pepper, deseeded and thinly sliced

1 small red onion, thinly sliced

2 garlic cloves, thinly sliced

100g/3½oz baby leaf spinach

200g/7oz canned chickpeas, drained and rinsed

2 tbsp 0% Greek yoghurt

2 tbsp reduced-fat guacamole

For the beetroot rice:

2 raw beetroot (beets), peeled and diced

1 tsp cumin seeds

a handful of dill or mint, chopped

grated zest and juice of 1 orange

1 tsp balsamic vinegar

30g/1oz reduced-fat feta cheese, crumbled

1 tsp toasted pine nuts

1 Put the prawns in a bowl with the lime juice, chilli and herbs. Season with black pepper and leave to marinate.

2 Make the beetroot rice: pulse the beetroot in a food processor or blender until it resembles small rice grains. Tip into a bowl and mix in the cumin seeds and most of the chopped herbs. Stir in the orange zest and juice and the vinegar, then sprinkle the feta and pine nuts over the top.

3 Lightly spray a large griddle or frying pan (skillet) with oil and set over a medium heat. Cook the green pepper, onion and garlic, stirring occasionally, for 6–8 minutes until tender. Add the spinach and chickpeas and cook for 1–2 minutes until the spinach wilts and turns bright green, and the chickpeas are hot. Remove the vegetables from the pan and keep warm.

4 Add the prawns in their marinade to the pan and cook for 2–3 minutes, turning occasionally, until uniformly pink.

5 Divide the beetroot rice between 2 serving plates and spoon the vegetable and chickpea mixture and prawns over the top. Serve with the yoghurt and guacamole.

CHEAT'S CHICKEN LASAGNE

This lasagne is really healthy and delicious and so much lower in calories than the traditional version made with sheets of pasta, white béchamel sauce and Parmesan. We have cheated and used thinly sliced pumpkin between the layers of sauce to add colour and natural sweetness. If fresh pumpkin's not available, use butternut squash instead – the calories will be about the same.

SERVES 2

Prep: 15 minutes

Cook: 45–50 mins

Per serving:

390 kcals

1632 kJ

5.5g fat

Low GI

low-cal spray oil

1 onion, diced

1 carrot, diced

100g/3½oz mushrooms, sliced

250g/9oz skinned chicken breast fillets, minced (ground)

1 x 400g/14oz can (scant 2 cups) chopped tomatoes

200g/7oz baby spinach leaves

sea salt and freshly ground black pepper

a few drops of balsamic vinegar

500g/1lb 2oz pumpkin

120g/4oz (½ cup) 0% fat Greek yoghurt

1 small free-range egg

> TIP: To ensure your chicken mince is fat-free, you can mince the skinned chicken breast fillets yourself, by pulsing in a blender or food processor.

1 Preheat the oven to 200°C, 400°F, gas 6.

2 Lightly spray a large deep frying pan (skillet) with oil and set over a medium heat. Cook the onion and carrot, stirring occasionally, for 6–8 minutes, until tender. Add the mushrooms and cook for 2–3 minutes until golden.

3 Stir in the chicken and cook, stirring, until lightly browned. Add the tomatoes and cook for about 5 minutes until reduced. Stir in the spinach and let it wilt into the mixture. Season to taste with salt and pepper and a few drops of balsamic vinegar.

4 Peel the pumpkin, discarding the seeds, and cut into very thin rounds or slices. A mandolin is best for this if you have one.

5 Cover the base of an ovenproof baking dish with a layer of overlapping pumpkin slices. Spoon over a layer of the chicken and tomato sauce. Continue layering up the dish in this way, finishing with a layer of sauce.

6 Beat together the Greek yoghurt and egg and pour over the top of the lasagne. Grind over a little black pepper and bake in the preheated oven for 25–30 minutes until bubbling and golden.

Amber option: If you want to make the topping crisp and cheesy, sprinkle the lasagne before cooking with 2 tbsp grated Parmesan and you will add 40 kcals and 2.9g fat per serving.

CHEAT'S CHICKEN TIKKA MASALA

Our cheat's chicken tikka masala is so much lower in calories and fat than the real version from an Indian restaurant or takeout, which can have as many as 680 kcals without rice. If served with pilau rice or naan bread, a single portion can be 1,000 kcals or more! We've used ground spices for speed but if you can grind them yourself with a pestle and mortar or spice grinder the flavour will be even better and more authentic.

SERVES 2

Prep: 15 minutes

Cook: 15 minutes

Per serving:

320 kcals

1339 kJ

3.5g fat

Low GI

1 small onion, diced

2 garlic cloves, crushed

1 green chilli, chopped

2.5cm/1in fresh root ginger, peeled and chopped

1 tsp ground turmeric

1 tsp ground coriander

½ tsp ground cumin

1 tsp garam masala

a small handful of coriander (cilantro) leaves, plus extra, chopped, to garnish

3 tbsp water

1 cinnamon stick

300g/10oz boned, skinned chicken breasts, cut into chunks

150ml/¼ pint (scant ¾ cup) vegetable stock

1 x 400g/14oz can (scant 2 cups) plum tomatoes

2 tbsp 0% fat Greek yoghurt

For the chilli broccoli:

4 spring onions (scallions), thinly sliced

a good pinch of cumin seeds

2 tbsp vegetable stock

150g/5oz broccoli, divided into florets

1 garlic clove, chopped

1 red chilli, deseeded and cut into fine shreds

sea salt and freshly ground black pepper

1 Put the onion, garlic, chilli, ginger, ground spices and coriander leaves in a blender or food processor, and blitz to a thick green paste. Add the water through the feed tube, a little at a time, to slacken it.

2 Cook the paste in a non-stick frying pan (skillet) set over a medium heat for 1 minute, stirring. Add the cinnamon stick and chicken and cook for 3 minutes, turning it in the spicy mixture.

3 Pour in the stock and tomatoes and reduce the heat to a simmer. Cover and cook gently for about 10 minutes or until the chicken is cooked through and tender. Discard the cinnamon stick.

4 Meanwhile, make the chilli broccoli: gently cook the spring onions, cumin seeds and stock in a pan set over a low heat for 5 minutes until the onions soften. Stir in the broccoli, garlic and chilli and cook for 5 minutes until the broccoli is tender. Season to taste with salt and plenty of black pepper.

5 Divide the chicken tikka masala between 2 serving plates. Top with the yoghurt and sprinkle with chopped coriander. Serve with the spicy broccoli.

Amber option: If you serve this with some plain boiled rice, a single portion of 30g/1oz (raw weight) will add 130 calories and 0.5g fat.

CHEAT'S 'PASTA'
with SOY *and* GARLIC CHICKEN DRUMSTICKS

SERVES 2

Prep: 10 minutes

Cook: 20 minutes

Per serving:

300 kcals

1255 kJ

5.5g fat

Low GI

Our 'pasta' is made with pretty green strands of low-calorie courgettes (zucchini). For the best results, you will need a spiraliser, julienne peeler or mandolin slicer but you can improvise with a potato peeler – just peel some long, thin lengths from the courgettes. You can make the chicken drumsticks stickier and sweeter if you add 2 teaspoons clear honey (21 extra kcals per serving) or 1 tablespoon sweet chilli sauce (17 extra kcals per serving) to the marinade coating.

2 large courgettes (zucchini), trimmed

low-cal spray oil

1 onion, finely chopped

a pinch of dried chilli flakes

juice of 2 lemons

120ml/4fl oz (½ cup) chicken stock

10 cherry tomatoes, quartered

1 small bunch of parsley, finely chopped

sea salt and freshly ground black pepper

lemon wedges, to garnish

For the chicken drumsticks:

4 x 125g/4oz skinned chicken drumsticks

3 tbsp dark soy sauce

a few drops of balsamic vinegar

2 garlic cloves, crushed

1 tsp grated fresh root ginger

1 Preheat the oven to 200°C, 400°F, gas mark 6.

2 Spiralise the courgettes lengthways, using blade C if you have a spiraliser. Alternatively, use a julienne peeler, mandolin slicer or even a potato peeler.

3 Put the chicken drumsticks in a dish. Mix together the soy sauce, balsamic vinegar, garlic and ginger, and spoon over the chicken, turning it until evenly coated. Transfer to an ovenproof dish or roasting pan and bake in the preheated oven for about 25–30 minutes until the chicken is cooked through.

4 Meanwhile, lightly spray a deep frying pan (skillet) with oil and set over a low to medium heat. Cook the onion, stirring occasionally, for 6–8 minutes until softened but not browned. Add the chilli flakes, lemon juice and stock and bring to the boil. Reduce the heat and stir in the tomatoes and half the parsley. Simmer gently for 5–10 minutes until the sauce reduces.

5 Add the spiralised courgettes and remaining parsley and cook for 1–2 minutes until the courgettes are just tender but still retain their shape – don't overcook them. Season to taste.

6 Serve immediately topped with the chicken drumsticks, with lemon wedges on the side.

CHEAT'S TANDOORI CHICKEN *with* CHANA DHAL

Instead of serving our low-fat tandoori chicken with pilau rice or naan bread, we've made some high-protein chana dhal with split chickpeas. It's a great source of dietary fibre and really fills you up, so you won't feel hungry. Don't be put off by the list of ingredients – this is really easy to make and you can prepare the chicken the night before and even make the dhal in advance to reheat later.

SERVES 2

Prep: 20 minutes

Chill: 1 hour minimum

Cook: 35–45 minutes

Per serving:

400 kcals

1674 kJ

6.2g fat

Low GI

2 tbsp tandoori paste

2 garlic cloves, crushed

1 tsp grated fresh root ginger

1 tsp paprika

½ tsp ground turmeric

juice of ½ lemon

60g/2oz (¼ cup) 0% fat Greek yoghurt

2 x 100g/3½oz skinned, boned chicken breasts

a handful of coriander (cilantro), chopped, to garnish

For the chana dhal:

100g/3½oz (½ cup) dried split chickpeas

480ml/16fl oz (2 cups) water

1 bay leaf

½ tsp ground coriander

½ tsp ground turmeric

½ tsp garam masala

a pinch of ground cardamom

1 tsp salt

For the carrot raita:

2 large carrots, coarsely grated

juice of 2 limes

a pinch of dried chilli flakes

1 tsp black mustard seeds

1 Stir together the tandoori paste, garlic, ginger, ground spices and lemon juice in a shallow bowl. Mix in the yoghurt.

2 Slash each chicken breast 3–4 times with a sharp knife and add to the marinade. Turn until well coated all over. Cover and chill in the fridge for at least 1 hour (or even overnight).

3 Make the chana dhal: put the split chickpeas and water in a large pan with the bay leaf, ground spices and salt. Bring to the boil, then reduce the heat and simmer, partially covered, for 30–40 minutes until the liquid is absorbed and the dhal is tender and moist. Check it occasionally: if it's too dry, add more water; too soupy, cook a little longer.

4 Meanwhile, make the carrot raita: mix the carrots, lime juice and chilli flakes in a bowl. Heat a frying pan (skillet) until it's really hot and cook the mustard seeds for 1–2 minutes, shaking gently, until they pop. Stir into the carrot mixture.

5 Preheat the oven to 220°C, 425°F, gas 7.

6 Remove the chicken from the marinade and transfer to a baking dish. Spoon the leftover marinade over the top. Bake in the preheated oven for 20 minutes, until the chicken is thoroughly cooked and slightly charred. Alternatively, cook under a hot grill (broiler), turning the breasts after 10 minutes to cook the other side.

7 Serve the tandoori chicken with the chana dhal, sprinkled with chopped coriander, with the carrot raita on the side.

CHEAT'S FISH *and* CHIPS

Battered fish and chips from a chip shop can contain as many as 800–1,000 kcals for an average portion, whereas our version has less than 300! Cod and haddock are the best fish to use as they keep their shape and don't fall apart. Be sure to use extra light (or lighter than light) mayo in the tartare sauce – only 10 kcals and 1g fat per tablespoon versus 35 kcals and 4g fat in light mayo.

SERVES 2

Prep: 15 minutes

Cook: 30–40 minutes

Per serving:

270 kcals

1130 kJ

4.3g fat

Low GI

low-cal spray oil

2 x 150g/5oz thick white fish fillets, pin-boned and skinned

a few sprigs of flat-leaf parsley, roughly chopped

1 lemon, cut into wedges

For the swede chips:

400g/14oz swede (rutabaga)

low-cal spray oil

1 tsp paprika

sea salt and freshly ground black pepper

For the tartare sauce:

150g/5oz (generous ½ cup) virtually fat-free fromage frais

2 tbsp extra light mayonnaise

2 tbsp chopped capers

2 small gherkins, diced

2 spring onions (scallions), diced

a few sprigs of dill, finely chopped

grated zest of ½ lemon and a squeeze of juice

1 Preheat the oven to 200°C, 400°F, gas 6.

2 Peel the swede and cut it into thin chips. Spread them out on a non-stick baking tray (cookie sheet) and lightly spray with oil. Dust with paprika and grind some sea salt and black pepper over the top.

3 Bake in the preheated oven for 30–40 minutes until the swede is cooked, crisp and golden brown.

4 About 15 minutes before the swede chips are ready, lightly spray a second baking tray with oil and place the fish fillets on it. Season with salt and pepper, then bake in the preheated oven for about 15 minutes until the fish is cooked and flakes easily. If it's getting a bit dry, cover with foil.

5 Meanwhile, make the tartare sauce: mix all the ingredients together in a bowl. Check the flavour and add some more lemon juice, a few drops of vinegar or salt and pepper if needed.

6 Serve the fish sprinkled with parsley, with the swede chips and tartare sauce. Squeeze the lemon wedges over the fish.

TIP: Vary the flavouring of the chips by dusting them with hot chilli powder, cayenne or even garam masala. Some garlic powder and a pinch of dried herbs are also good.

CHICKEN PASTA BAKE

This delicious bake topped with melted mozzarella cheese will fill you up and prevent those hunger pangs that can trigger snacking. You can vary the vegetables and use green or red (bell) peppers or an aubergine (eggplant) without affecting the overall calorie count.

....

SERVES 2

Prep: 15 minutes

Cook: 35–40 minutes

Per serving:

430 kcals

1799 kJ

5.7g fat

Medium GI

100g/3½oz penne or macaroni (dry weight)

low-cal spray oil

1 small red onion, diced

1 yellow (bell) pepper, deseeded and cut into chunks

1 large courgette (zucchini), thickly sliced

200g/7oz skinned chicken breast fillets, cubed

1 x 200g/7oz can (scant 1 cup) chopped tomatoes

1 tbsp tomato paste

a few basil leaves, torn

sea salt and freshly ground black pepper

60g/2oz reduced-fat mozzarella, torn into pieces

balsamic vinegar for drizzling (optional)

1 Preheat the oven to 200°C, 400°F, gas mark 6.

2 Cook the pasta according to the instructions on the packet and drain well.

3 Meanwhile, lightly spray a large frying pan (skillet) with oil and set over a low to medium heat. Cook the onion, yellow pepper and courgette for 4–5 minutes until starting to soften. Add the chicken and cook for 5 minutes, turning occasionally, until golden.

4 Add the tomatoes, tomato paste and basil leaves and simmer gently for 8–10 minutes until reduced and thickened. Season with salt and pepper to taste.

5 Stir the pasta into the chicken and vegetables and spoon into a shallow ovenproof dish. Sprinkle the mozzarella over the top and bake in the preheated oven for 15–20 minutes until bubbling and golden brown on top.

6 Serve immediately, drizzled with balsamic vinegar (if using), with a salad from the 'green' list.

CHICKEN SALTIMBOCCA *with* LEMONY SMASHED PESTO POTATOES

SERVES 2

Prep: 10 minutes

Cook: 25 minutes

Per serving:

410 kcals

1715 kJ

10.5g fat

Medium GI

Saltimbocca makes a really quick and simple supper when you don't have much time to cook. If wished, you can substitute turkey breast or veal escalopes (cutlets) for the chicken and 0% fat Greek yoghurt for the crème fraîche. The calories will stay approximately the same.

2 x 100g/3½oz skinned, boned chicken breasts

4 sage leaves

4 thin slices lean Parma ham, all visible fat removed

low-cal spray oil

200g/7oz button mushrooms, thinly sliced

210ml/7fl oz (scant 1 cup) chicken stock

60ml/2fl oz (¼ cup) Marsala

sea salt and freshly ground black pepper

2 tbsp half-fat crème fraîche

300g/10oz small new potatoes, scrubbed

grated zest and juice of 1 small lemon

1 tbsp green pesto

a handful of parsley, chopped

1 Place each chicken breast between 2 sheets of parchment paper or cling film (plastic wrap) and beat with a rolling pin until thin and flat like an escalope (cutlet).

2 Place 2 sage leaves on top of each chicken escalope and wrap 2 slices of Parma ham around each.

3 Lightly spray a large frying pan (skillet) with oil and set over a medium heat. Add the chicken to the hot pan and cook for 4–5 minutes until golden brown on both sides. Add the mushrooms and cook for 3–4 minutes, stirring occasionally, until lightly browned.

4 Add the chicken stock and Marsala and reduce the heat to low. Simmer gently for about 10 minutes until the chicken is cooked right through and the sauce is reduced and syrupy. Season to taste with salt and pepper, then stir in the crème fraîche. Heat through very gently without boiling.

5 While the chicken's cooking, cook the potatoes in a pan of lightly salted boiling water for about 15 minutes until tender. Drain well and then return to the hot pan with the lemon zest and juice and pesto. Lightly mash the potatoes with a fork, not too much – they should stay reasonably chunky but mashed round the edges.

6 Serve the saltimbocca sprinkled with parsley, with the smashed pesto potatoes.

TIP: Marsala is a sweet-tasting fortified wine from Sicily. You can buy it in most supermarkets and off-licences (liquor stores).

THAI GREEN PRAWN *and* COCONUT CURRY

SERVES 2

Prep: 10 minutes

Cook: 20 minutes

This aromatic curry is easy to make and fills you up. If wished, you can use 200g/7oz skinned chicken breast fillet instead of prawns (shrimp) and you will have 450 kcals and 11g fat per serving. Add the chicken with the aubergine (eggplant) and cook as instructed.

Per serving:

420 kcals

9.7g fat

Medium GI

low-cal spray oil

1 red onion, diced

2 garlic cloves, crushed

2.5cm/1in fresh root ginger, peeled and chopped

1 aubergine (eggplant), cubed

2 tbsp Thai green curry paste

150g/5oz cherry tomatoes, halved

150ml/¼ pint (generous ½ cup) reduced-fat coconut milk

1 tbsp nam pla (Thai fish sauce)

200g/7oz peeled raw tiger prawns (shrimp)

a handful of coriander (cilantro), chopped

100g/3½oz (scant ½ cup) basmati rice (dry weight)

a few basil leaves, shredded

1 Lightly spray a large non-stick frying pan (skillet) with oil and set over a medium heat. Add the onion, garlic and ginger and cook, stirring occasionally, for 5 minutes until golden and tender.

2 Add the aubergine and cook gently, stirring occasionally, for 3–4 minutes until tender and golden brown all over.

3 Stir in the curry paste and cook for 1 minute, then add the tomatoes and cook for 2 minutes. Pour in the coconut milk and nam pla, and cook gently for a few minutes until the sauce starts to thicken and reduce slightly.

4 Stir in the prawns and cook, turning them once or twice, for 2–3 minutes until pink on both sides. Stir in the coriander.

5 Meanwhile, steam or boil the rice according to the instructions on the packet.

6 Divide the prawn curry between two serving plates and serve with the rice. Scatter the basil leaves over the top.

> TIP: You can use Thai red curry paste instead of green without changing the calories and fat grams per portion.

SHRIMP SCAMPI

This is a traditional Sicilian dish. If you love garlic you can add some extra cloves for approximately the same calories. You don't need fresh shellfish – just use the packs of frozen tiger prawns (shrimp) from the freezer aisle in your local supermarket. Be sure to defrost them thoroughly before cooking. If wished, you can serve this with rocket (arugula) or stir a handful into the pan just before serving. This adds about 5 kcals per serving.

SERVES 2

Prep: 5 minutes

Cook: 10 minutes

Per serving:

440 kcals

1841 kJ

2.2g fat

Low GI

150g/5oz spaghetti or linguine (dry weight)

sea salt and freshly ground black pepper

low-cal spray oil

3 garlic cloves, crushed

a pinch of dried chilli flakes

1 bunch of parsley, finely chopped

1 small bunch of chives, snipped

juice of 1 large lemon

120ml/4fl oz (½ cup) dry white wine

2 tomatoes, diced

250g/9oz peeled raw tiger prawns (shrimp)

1 Cook the pasta in a large pan of boiling salted water according to the instructions on the packet, until just tender (*al dente*). Drain well.

2 Meanwhile, lightly spray a large deep frying pan (skillet) with oil and set over a medium heat. Add the garlic and cook for 1 minute without colouring. Stir in the chilli flakes and half of the herbs, then pour in the lemon juice and wine and bring to the boil. Let it bubble away for 4–5 minutes until the liquid reduces.

3 Add the tomatoes and prawns and cook, turning once, for about 2 minutes until the prawns are pink on both sides. Season to taste with salt and pepper, and stir in the remaining herbs.

4 Add the drained pasta to the pan and toss lightly together until all the strands are coated with the sauce.

5 Divide the pasta between 2 shallow serving bowls and serve immediately.

CRISPY BAKED SALMON *and* SPINACH

SERVES 2

Prep: 10 minutes

Cook: 50 minutes

This crispy bake is really delicious, healthy and packed with nutrients. Salmon, like other oily fish, is a great source of omega-3 oils, which are beneficial for your cardiovascular health. This is a low-fat way to make a white sauce – you can use this method when making cauliflower gratin, macaroni cheese or a lasagne.

Per serving:

450 kcals

1883 kJ

13g fat

Medium GI

250g/9oz potatoes, peeled

200g/7oz baby spinach leaves

200g/7oz skinned salmon fillets, cut into large chunks

1 bunch of chives, finely chopped

For the white sauce:

2 tbsp cornflour (cornstarch)

300ml/½ pint (1¼ cups) skimmed milk

2 tbsp virtually fat-free fromage frais

a pinch of ground nutmeg

grated zest of 1 lemon

sea salt and freshly ground black pepper

1 Preheat the oven to 200°C, 400°F, gas mark 6.

2 Cook the potatoes in a pan of boiling salted water for 10–12 minutes until just tender but still firm and not falling apart. Drain and cool, then cut lengthways into thin slices.

3 Put the spinach in a bowl and pour some boiling water over it. Tip into a colander and drain well, pressing out the excess water with a saucer. Put the spinach and salmon in an ovenproof baking dish. Sprinkle the chives over the top.

4 Make the white sauce: stir the cornflour into a little of the milk to make a smooth paste. Heat the remaining milk in a pan and, as soon as it starts to boil, reduce the heat and stir in the cornflour mixture. Cook gently, stirring with a wooden spoon for 2–3 minutes until the sauce is thick and smooth and coats the back of the spoon. Remove from the heat and stir in the fromage frais, nutmeg and lemon zest. Season to taste.

5 Pour the white sauce over the salmon and spinach and arrange the potatoes in overlapping slices over the top so everything is completely covered.

6 Bake in the preheated oven for about 30 minutes until the salmon is cooked through, the sauce is bubbling and the potato topping is golden brown and crisp.

JAPANESE GRIDDLED TUNA STEAKS *and* BROWN RICE

SERVES 2

Prep: 15 minutes

Cook: 20 minutes

Per serving:

450 kcals

1883 kJ

8.3g fat

Medium GI

Fresh tuna is a good source of omega-3 oil for heart health. It's lower in fat and calories than salmon and much more 'meaty'. You can buy packs of sprouted alfalfa seeds in most supermarkets and health food stores, or try sprouting them yourself at home to add to salads.

100g/3½oz (scant ½ cup) brown rice (dry weight)

80g/3oz (1 cup) sprouted seeds, e.g. alfalfa

1 tbsp black or white sesame seeds

1 tbsp teriyaki sauce

2 x 125g/4oz fresh tuna steaks

low-cal spray oil

For the dressing:

1 tbsp miso paste

1 tbsp rice vinegar or mirin

1 tbsp soy sauce

grated zest and juice of 2 limes

2 tsp grated fresh root ginger

1 tsp sugar

1 Cook the brown rice according to the instructions on the packet. Drain and transfer to a large bowl. Leave to cool.

2 Make the dressing: whisk all the ingredients together until well blended, or shake vigorously in a screw-top jar.

3 Stir the rice with a fork to separate the grains and gently mix in the sprouted seeds. Add most of the dressing and stir into the rice.

4 Toast the sesame seeds in a small dry frying pan (skillet) set over a medium to high heat for 1–2 minutes until they release their aroma. Don't let them burn. Remove from the pan and set aside to cool.

5 Put the teriyaki sauce in a bowl and add the tuna, turning it until coated in the sauce. Lightly spray a non-stick griddle pan with oil and set over a medium to high heat. Cook the tuna steaks for 2–4 minutes each side, depending on how well done you like them. Remove from the pan and cut into slices.

6 Divide the rice salad between 2 serving plates and top with the sliced tuna. Drizzle with the remaining dressing and sprinkle with the sesame seeds.

CHEAT'S SWEET *and* SOUR PORK

The real thing from a Chinese restaurant or takeout can be horrendously high in calories and fat as the pork is usually deep-fried in batter. It usually averages 700–800 kcals per serving, including plain boiled rice. Our version is much healthier and more slimming and it's really quick and easy to make, too.

SERVES 2

Prep: 15 minutes

Cook: 8 minutes

Per serving:

420 kcals

1757 kJ

3.3g fat

Medium GI

low-cal spray oil

200g/7oz lean pork fillet (all visible fat removed), cubed

2 garlic cloves, crushed

4 spring onions (scallions), sliced diagonally

1 green (bell) pepper, deseeded and cut into chunks

1 red (bell) pepper, deseeded and cut into chunks

2 canned pineapple slices in natural juice, cut into chunks

sea salt and freshly ground black pepper

100g/3½oz (scant ½ cup) basmati rice (dry weight)

For the sweet and sour sauce:

1 tbsp white wine vinegar

2 tbsp soy sauce

1 tbsp tomato paste

1 tbsp sherry or rice wine

juice of 1 large orange

1 tsp brown sugar

1 tbsp cornflour (cornstarch)

1 Make the sweet and sour sauce: mix all the ingredients together in a bowl until really smooth and there are no lumps.

2 Lightly spray a wok or deep frying pan (skillet) with oil and set over a medium to high heat. When it's very hot, add the pork and stir-fry for 5 minutes until it's cooked right through and golden brown all over.

3 Add the garlic, spring onions and peppers and stir-fry for 2–3 minutes.

4 Add the pineapple and the sweet and sour sauce. Keep stirring for 1–2 minutes until the sauce thickens and coats the pork and vegetables. Season to taste with salt and pepper.

5 Meanwhile, cook the rice according to the instructions on the packet.

6 Divide the rice between two serving plates and serve the sweet and sour pork on top.

SPICY STIR-FRIED QUINOA

The beauty of this dish is that it can be eaten hot or cold. You could even put a portion in a container and take it to work or college as a packed lunch. Serve it with sweet chilli sauce and you'll add about 30 kcals per tablespoon.

SERVES 2

Prep: 15 minutes

Cook: 20 minutes

Per serving:

370 kcals

1548 kJ

11g fat

Low GI

25g/1oz cashews

240ml/8fl oz (1 cup) vegetable stock

100g/3½oz (generous ½ cup) quinoa (dry weight)

150g/5oz broccoli, separated into florets

100g/3½oz mange tout (snow peas), trimmed

low-cal spray oil

4 spring onions (scallions), sliced

1 red (bell) pepper, deseeded and diced

2 garlic cloves, crushed

2.5cm/1in fresh root ginger, peeled and diced

1 red chilli, cut into fine shreds

½ tsp ground coriander

2 tbsp light soy sauce

grated zest and juice of 1 lime

100g/3½oz baby plum tomatoes, quartered

sea salt and freshly ground black pepper

a handful of coriander (cilantro), chopped

1 Set a small dry frying pan (skillet) over a medium heat. Add the cashews to the hot pan, gently tossing and turning them, for 1–2 minutes until golden brown. Remove from the heat immediately before they catch and burn, and tip onto a plate. Set aside to cool.

2 Heat the stock in a pan and, when it starts to boil, add the quinoa. Cover and simmer gently for 15 minutes until tender and most of the liquid has been absorbed. The quinoa is cooked when the 'sprout' pops out of the seed. Take off the heat and leave to steam in the pan for 5 minutes or so before draining off any liquid. Fluff up the quinoa with a fork.

3 Meanwhile, blanch the broccoli in a pan of boiling water for 1 minute. Plunge into a bowl of iced water to cool, then drain and set aside. Repeat with the mange tout.

4 Lightly spray a wok or frying pan with oil and stir-fry the spring onions, red pepper, garlic, ginger and chilli over a medium heat for 2 minutes. Stir in the ground coriander, soy sauce, lime zest and juice, broccoli, mange tout and tomatoes. Stir-fry for 1–2 minutes. Add the drained quinoa and heat through for 1 minute. Season with salt and pepper to taste.

5 Divide between 2 shallow bowls and sprinkle the toasted cashews and coriander over the top. Serve immediately.

CHEAT'S SPAGHETTI BOLOGNESE

Our cheat's spaghetti bolognese uses mushrooms instead of minced beef. If you use 200g/7oz extra lean minced (ground) beef (less than 5% fat) instead, you will increase the kcals per serving to 500 plus an extra 5g fat. Don't be tempted to sprinkle the finished dish with more cheese – a single tablespoon is 40 kcals and 3g fat.

SERVES 2

Prep: 10 minutes

Cook: 25 minutes

Per serving:

390 kcals

1632 kJ

3.7g fat

Low GI

low-cal spray oil

1 large onion, diced

2 garlic cloves, crushed

400g/14oz firm mushrooms, quartered

150ml/¼ pint (generous ½ cup) stock made with a porcini stock cube

1 x 400g/14oz can (scant 2 cups) chopped tomatoes

1 tbsp tomato paste

a few basil leaves, torn

a few drops of balsamic vinegar (optional)

sea salt and freshly ground black pepper

150g/5oz spaghetti (dry weight)

1 tbsp grated Parmesan cheese

1 Lightly spray a large saucepan with oil and set over a low heat. Gently cook the onion and garlic, stirring occasionally, for 8–10 minutes until tender and golden but not browned.

2 Add the mushrooms and cook for about 5 minutes, stirring occasionally, until golden. Add the stock, tomatoes and tomato paste. Bring to the boil, then reduce the heat and simmer gently for about 10 minutes until the sauce reduces and thickens. Stir in the basil and balsamic vinegar (if using) and season to taste.

3 Meanwhile, cook the spaghetti in a large pan of boiling salted water according to the packet instructions until just tender (al dente). Drain well.

4 Toss the spaghetti in the mushroom sauce and divide between 2 serving plates. Sprinkle with Parmesan and serve immediately.

> TIP: If you don't have a porcini mushroom stock cube, just use a vegetable stock cube or bouillon powder instead.

CHEAT'S CHILLI CON CARNE

You can make this a day ahead and keep it covered in the fridge overnight to reheat the following day. It also freezes well. We've served our version with quinoa, which is highly nutritious and a good source of protein, dietary fibre, vitamins and minerals.

....

SERVES 2

Prep: 10 minutes

Cook: 40–45 minutes

Per serving:

440 kcals

1841 kJ

9g fat

Low GI

low-cal spray oil

1 small red onion, diced

1 red (bell) pepper, deseeded and chopped

1 red chilli, diced

200g/7oz (scant 1 cup) extra lean minced (ground) beef (max 5% fat)

1 tsp cumin seeds

1 tsp ground cinnamon

1 tsp chilli powder

1 x 400g/14oz can (scant 2 cups) chopped tomatoes

240ml/8fl oz (1 cup) beef stock

100g/3½oz (1¾ cups) canned kidney beans, rinsed and drained

sea salt and freshly ground black pepper

80g/3oz (½ cup) quinoa (dry weight)

a handful of coriander (cilantro), roughly chopped

2 tbsp 0% fat Greek yoghurt

1 Lightly spray a large pan with oil and set over a low to medium heat. Cook the onion, red pepper and chilli, stirring occasionally, for about 8–10 minutes until softened.

2 Add the minced beef, cumin seeds, cinnamon and chilli powder. Cook for 5 minutes, stirring occasionally, until the mince is browned all over.

3 Add the tomatoes and stock and simmer gently for 20–30 minutes until the sauce reduces and thickens. Stir in the kidney beans and cook for 2–3 minutes to warm them through. Season to taste with salt and pepper.

4 Meanwhile, cook the quinoa according to the instructions on the packet.

5 Divide the quinoa between 2 serving plates and top with the chilli. Sprinkle with coriander and serve with a spoonful of yoghurt.

CHEAT'S PAD THAI

If you eat this in a Thai restaurant or order a takeout, a typical single portion of pad Thai may contain approximately 600 kcals (some as much as 900!). Don't be tempted to add more peanuts – every nut has an amazing 6 kcals and 0.5g fat, so it's easy to see how quickly they add up.

SERVES 2

Prep: 10 minutes

Cook: 6–8 minutes

Per serving:

390 kcals

1632 kJ

8.5g fat

Medium GI

100g/3½oz flat rice noodles (dry weight)

low-cal spray oil

2 garlic cloves, crushed

4 spring onions (scallions), sliced

1 red chilli, diced

200g/7oz peeled raw prawns (shrimp)

1 medium free-range egg, lightly beaten

grated zest and juice of 1 lime

2 tbsp nam pla (Thai fish sauce)

1 tbsp soy sauce

1 tsp brown sugar

100g/3½oz (1 cup) bean sprouts

15g/½oz unsalted roasted peanuts

a handful of coriander (cilantro), chopped

1 Prepare the rice noodles according to the instructions on the packet.

2 Lightly spray a wok or deep frying pan (skillet) with oil and set over a high heat. Add the garlic, spring onions and chilli and stir-fry for 1 minute. Add the prawns and stir-fry for 1 minute.

3 Add the drained rice noodles and stir-fry for 2 minutes. Push everything to the side and add the beaten egg. Cook for 1 minute, stirring all the time, until it scrambles. Stir into the noodle mixture.

4 Add the lime zest and juice, nam pla, soy sauce, brown sugar and bean sprouts. Stir-fry for 1 minute.

5 Finally, stir in the peanuts and coriander and remove from the heat. Divide between 2 shallow serving bowls and eat immediately.

CHEAT'S SEAFOOD RISOTTO

SERVES 2

Prep: 10 minutes

Cook: 30 minutes

Per serving:

390 kcals

1632 kJ

3.5g fat

Medium GI

Most supermarkets sell packs of frozen seafood (fruits de mer), which contain mixed prawns (shrimp), mussels and squid. Or you can use frozen jumbo prawns without affecting the overall calorie count. Be careful to defrost them thoroughly before use. The secret to a good risotto is patience: keep the stock simmering in a hot pan on the stove and add it a ladleful at a time. Keep stirring until it's absorbed before adding more.

low-cal spray oil

1 onion, finely chopped

2 garlic cloves, crushed

a good pinch of chilli powder

100g/3½oz (scant ½ cup) risotto rice, e.g. Arborio, Carnaroli (dry weight)

120ml/4fl oz (½ cup) dry white wine or vermouth

480ml/16fl oz (2 cups) hot chicken or fish stock

a pinch of saffron threads

100g/3½oz cherry tomatoes, halved

300g/10oz frozen seafood, defrosted

juice of 1 lemon

1 small bunch of parsley, chopped

sea salt and freshly ground black pepper

1 Lightly spray a large deep frying pan (skillet) with oil and set over a low heat. Cook the onion and garlic, stirring occasionally, for about 10 minutes until tender but not coloured.

2 Stir in the chilli powder and the rice, then cook for 1 minute. Pour in the wine or vermouth and cook over a medium heat until all the liquid has almost evaporated.

3 Reduce the heat to a gentle simmer and add a ladle of hot stock together with the saffron. Stir gently with a wooden spoon and when it's absorbed, add another ladleful. Keep doing this, stirring with each addition until all the liquid has been absorbed and the rice is cooked and tender. It should be al dente (still retain some 'bite') rather than mushy.

4 Stir in the tomatoes and seafood. Cook for 3–4 minutes over a low heat until the prawns are pink on both sides. Stir in the lemon juice and parsley and season to taste with salt and pepper.

5 Spoon the risotto into 2 shallow serving dishes and enjoy.

> TIP: In Italy, seafood risotto is never served with cheese. If you choose to sprinkle 1 tablespoon of grated Parmesan over each serving you will add 40 kcals and 3g fat.

CHEAT'S MACARONI CHEESE

This low-calorie deluxe version of that old favourite macaroni cheese tastes fabulous as well as delivering a good portion of your 5-a-day vegetables. You can use any pasta shapes – penne (tubes), fusilli (spirals) or conchiglie (shells) also work well.

SERVES 2

Prep: 10 minutes

Cook: 25–30 minutes

Per serving:

400 kcals

1674 kJ

4.8g fat

Medium GI

100g/3½oz (1 cup) macaroni (dry weight)

low-cal spray oil

1 large leek, trimmed and sliced

200g/7oz button mushrooms, quartered

12 baby plum tomatoes, halved

a handful of parsley, chopped

1 tbsp grated half-fat Cheddar cheese

2 tbsp fresh white or wholemeal breadcrumbs

For the white sauce:

2 tbsp cornflour (cornstarch)

300ml/½ pint (1¼ cups) skimmed milk

2 tbsp virtually fat-free fromage frais

a pinch of ground nutmeg

grated zest of 1 lemon

sea salt and freshly ground black pepper

1 Preheat the oven to 190°C, 375°F, gas mark 5.

2 Cook the macaroni in a large pan of lightly salted boiling water according to the packet instructions. Drain and keep warm.

3 Meanwhile, make the white sauce: stir the cornflour into a little of the milk to make a smooth paste. Heat the remaining milk in a pan and, as soon as it starts to boil, reduce the heat and stir in the cornflour mixture. Cook gently, stirring with a wooden spoon for 2–3 minutes until the sauce is thick and smooth and coats the back of the spoon. Remove from the heat and stir in the fromage frais, nutmeg and lemon zest. Season to taste with salt and pepper.

4 Lightly spray a pan with oil and set over a low heat. Add the leek and mushrooms and cook gently for 5 minutes until softened. Stir in the tomatoes and parsley and cook for 1 minute.

5 Combine the macaroni and the leek and mushroom mixture in an ovenproof dish. Pour over the white sauce and sprinkle with the grated cheese and breadcrumbs.

6 Bake in the preheated oven for 15–20 minutes, until bubbling and golden brown. Serve immediately.

SKINNY LASAGNE STACKS

This lasagne is made in individual portions without white sauce. Choose really lean minced (ground) good-quality beef with less than 5% fat. You can make double the quantity if wished and then cool and freeze the extra portions to be defrosted and reheated at a later date.

SERVES 2

Prep: 10 minutes

Cook: 1 hour

Per serving:

405 kcals

1548 kJ

7g fat

Low GI

low-cal spray oil

1 small onion, chopped

2 garlic cloves, crushed

1 carrot, diced

1 celery stick, diced

200g/7oz extra lean minced (ground) beef (max. 5% fat)

1 tbsp tomato paste

90ml/3fl oz (scant ½ cup) red wine

120ml/4fl oz (½ cup) skimmed milk

1 x 200g/7oz can (scant 1 cup) chopped tomatoes

1 bay leaf

a few sprigs of thyme

sea salt and freshly ground black pepper

4 lasagne sheets

2 tbsp low-fat crème fraîche

2 tsp grated Parmesan cheese

1 Lightly spray a saucepan with oil and set over a low to medium heat. Cook the onion, garlic, carrot and celery, stirring occasionally, for about 6–8 minutes until softened. Add the mince and cook, stirring, for 4–5 minutes until browned all over.

2 Stir in the tomato paste, wine and milk and bring to the boil. Reduce the heat and add the tomatoes, herbs and salt and pepper to taste. Simmer gently for 30–40 minutes until the sauce has reduced and there's no more liquid. Remove the bay leaf and thyme stalks.

3 Cook the lasagne sheets in a large pan of boiling salted water, according to the packet instructions, and drain well.

4 Preheat the overhead grill (broiler) and line the grill pan with a sheet of kitchen foil.

5 Place 2 sheets of lasagne on the lined grill pan. Spoon the sauce over the top and cover with the remaining sheets of lasagne. Smear the crème fraîche over the top and sprinkle with the Parmesan. Pop under the hot grill for a few minutes – just long enough to melt the cheese and brown the top.

6 Use a large slice to transfer the lasagne stacks to 2 serving plates, and eat with green vegetables or a salad from the 'green' list (page 11).

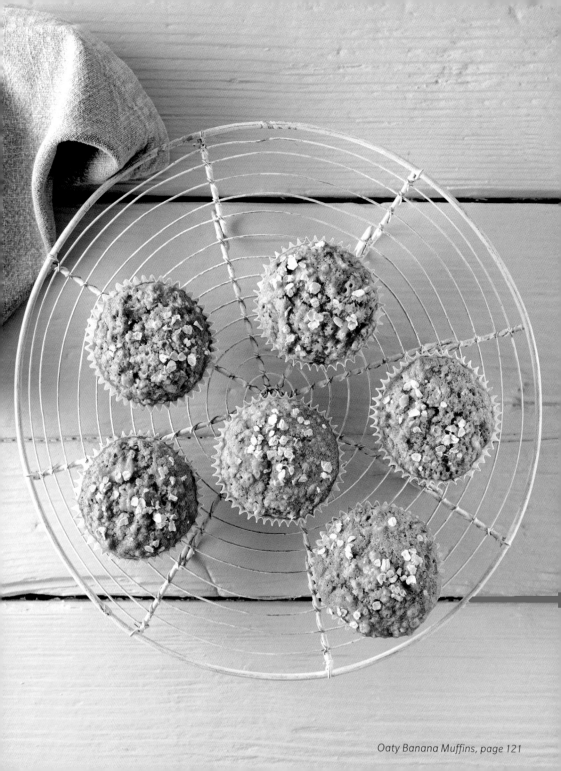

Oaty Banana Muffins, page 121

Treat yourself

(snacks & desserts)

SNACKS (MAX 100 KCALS)

Cheat's butternut squash 'fries'

Roasted vegetable wedges with tzatziki

Cheat's buffalo wings

Cheat's hummus

Prawn, mango and avocado wraps

Italian tricolore kebabs

CAKES & DESSERTS (MAX 200 KCALS)

Passionfruit mini pavlovas

Affogato

Frozen yoghurt strawberries

Strawberry and lemon curd meringue mess

Fruit kebabs with chocolate sauce

Peachy chocolate filo parcels

Oaty banana muffins

Cheat's tiramisu

Cheat's low-fat carrot cake

Cheat's brownies

Cheat's espresso chocolate mousse

Cheat's apple crumble

CHEAT'S BUTTERNUT SQUASH 'FRIES'

Our cheat's 'fries' have a fraction of the fat and calories in French fries, and they're easy to make and taste delicious. You can use ready-made seasoning if you don't want to mix your own – buy a small jar of Cajun, harissa, ras-el-hanout, fajita or jerk seasoning.

SERVES 2

Prep: 15 minutes

Cook: 20–30 mins

Per serving:

100 kcals

418 kJ

0.6g fat

Low GI

1 x 300g/10oz butternut squash

1 tsp black peppercorns

1 tsp paprika

½ tsp garlic powder

a good pinch of chilli powder

1 tsp dried mixed herbs

low-cal spray oil

For the fruity salsa:

2 ripe tomatoes, diced

1 red chilli, diced

½ red (bell) pepper, deseeded and diced

¼ red onion, diced

1 juicy small peach, stoned (pitted) and diced

a few sprigs of coriander (cilantro), chopped

sea salt and freshly ground black pepper

1 Preheat the oven to 200°C, 400°F, gas mark 6.

2 Peel the butternut squash, then cut in half and scoop out and discard the seeds. Cut the orange flesh into thin strips and arrange on a non-stick baking tray (cookie sheet).

3 Grind the black peppercorns in a pepper grinder or with a pestle and mortar and mix with the paprika, garlic powder, chilli powder and herbs.

4 Lightly spray the butternut squash with oil and sprinkle with the spicy seasoning mixture. Bake in the preheated oven for 20–30 minutes until crisp and golden brown.

5 Meanwhile, make the fruity salsa: mix all the ingredients together in a bowl and season to taste.

6 Serve the hot butternut squash 'fries' immediately with the salsa.

ROASTED VEGETABLE WEDGES *with* TZATZIKI

SERVES 2

Prep: 10 minutes

Cook: 20–25 mins

Roasted vegetables are surprisingly filling and a very healthy snack. You can use virtually any vegetables on the 'green' list, depending on the season and what you've got available. Try chunks of leeks, asparagus, carrots, swede (rutabaga), pumpkin, butternut squash and onion wedges.

Per serving:

100 kcals

418 kJ

1.2g fat

Low GI

1 large courgette (zucchini), cut into chunks

1 red (bell) pepper, deseeded and cut into chunks

1 aubergine (eggplant), cut into chunks

low-cal spray oil

a few sprigs of rosemary and thyme

sea salt and freshly ground black pepper

For the tzatziki:

120g/4oz (generous ½ cup) 0% fat Greek yoghurt

¼ cucumber, diced

1 garlic clove, crushed

a squeeze of lemon juice

a handful of mint, chopped

a handful of dill or flat-leaf parsley, chopped

1 Preheat the oven to 200°C, 400°F, gas mark 6.

2 Arrange the vegetable chunks on a non-stick baking tray (cookie sheet) and lightly spray with oil. Strip the leaves from the rosemary and thyme sprigs and sprinkle over the top. Give everything a good grinding of salt and black pepper.

3 Cook in the preheated oven for 20–25 minutes until the vegetables are tender and just starting to colour and char around the edges.

4 Meanwhile, make the tzatziki: mix all the ingredients together in a bowl.

5 Serve the roasted vegetables, hot or cold, with the tzatziki dip.

CHEAT'S BUFFALO WINGS

You can buy ready-prepared chicken wings or ask your butcher to do it for you. As an alternative dip, just stir some chopped herbs and crushed garlic into the yoghurt.

SERVES 2

Prep: 10 minutes

Chill: 30 minutes

Cook: 12–15 mins

Per serving:

100 kcals

418 kJ

2.5g fat

Low GI

1 tsp hoisin sauce

2 tsp dark soy sauce

½ tsp sweet chilli sauce

1 tsp tomato ketchup

1 garlic clove, crushed

grated zest and juice of ½ orange

3 x 85g/3oz chicken wings, skinned and cut in 2

For the honey mustard dip:

60g/2oz (¼ cup) 0% fat Greek yoghurt

1 tsp honey mustard

1 Make the honey mustard dip: mix the yoghurt and honey mustard in a small bowl. Cover and leave to chill in the fridge.

2 Mix together the hoisin, soy and sweet chilli sauces with the tomato ketchup, garlic, orange zest and juice in a larger bowl. Add the chicken wings and turn them in the marinade until coated all over. Cover with cling film (plastic wrap) and chill in the fridge for at least 30 minutes.

3 Preheat an overhead grill (broiler) until it's very hot.

4 Place the chicken wings in a foil-lined grill pan and spoon any remaining marinade over the top. Cook under the preheated grill for 12–15 minutes, turning occasionally and basting with the marinade, until crisp and sticky and cooked right through.

5 Serve the hot chicken wings immediately with the honey mustard dip on the side.

CHEAT'S HUMMUS

The hummus you buy in the supermarket or deli can be very high in calories and fat – you even need to check the labels of the low-fat versions carefully. This cheat's hummus is so simple to make and tastes great with vegetable dippers or spread on a crispbread or rice cake.

SERVES 3

Prep: 10 minutes

Per serving:

100 kcals

418 kJ

4g fat

Low GI

1 x 200g/7oz (¾ cup)can chickpeas

2 garlic cloves, crushed

1 tsp tahini

juice of ½ lemon

½ tsp ground cumin

2 tbsp 0% fat Greek yoghurt

sea salt and freshly ground black pepper

cayenne for dusting

1 Drain the chickpeas, reserving the liquid. Rinse the chickpeas in a sieve under cold running water and drain well.

2 Put the chickpeas, garlic, tahini, lemon juice and cumin in a blender and blitz until you have a thick, slightly grainy purée.

3 If necessary, thin it a little with 1–2 tablespoons of the reserved chickpea liquid. It should have the consistency of thick cream.

4 Transfer the hummus to a serving bowl and stir in the yoghurt. Season to taste with salt and pepper. Dust lightly with cayenne. This will keep, covered, in the fridge for 2–3 days.

> **TIP:** You can flavour the hummus with chopped herbs, such as chives, coriander (cilantro) or parsley, or a diced red chilli. The calorie count will stay roughly the same.

PRAWN, MANGO *and* AVOCADO WRAPS

These healthy low-fat 'wraps' are made with large crisp iceberg lettuce leaves rather than high-calorie tortillas. You can vary the filling according to preference and what you've got in your fridge or store cupboard. Try cooked chicken, drained canned beans or chickpeas, reduced-fat hummus, tzatziki, cottage cheese, papaya, peaches – there are so many delicious possibilities.

SERVES 2

Prep: 10 minutes

Per serving:

100 kcals

418 kJ

0.7g fat

Low GI

½ ripe mango

100g/3½oz cooked peeled prawns (shrimp)

1 small bunch of chives, snipped

2 tbsp 0% fat Greek yoghurt

2 tsp extra light mayonnaise

grated zest and juice of ½ lime

sea salt and freshly ground black pepper

2 large iceberg lettuce leaves

1 tbsp sweet chilli sauce

1 Remove the skin and stone from the mango and cut the flesh into dice. Mix the mango, prawns and chives together in a bowl.

2 Blend the yoghurt and mayonnaise with the lime zest and juice. Stir into the prawn and mango mixture. Season lightly with salt and pepper.

3 Place the iceberg lettuce leaves on a clean board or work surface and divide the prawn and mango mixture between them. Drizzle with the chilli sauce.

4 Fold the sides of the lettuce leaves over the filling into the centre, and then fold the ends over to completely enclose the filling and make 2 neat parcels. Alternatively, just roll up the lettuce leaves around the filling, like a cigar.

5 If you're not going to eat them straight away, wrap in cling film (plastic wrap) and chill in the fridge for up to a few hours – not too long or the lettuce will start to lose its crispness and go soggy.

ITALIAN TRICOLORE KEBABS

These snacks can also be served as canapés at parties or with pre-dinner drinks. Choose an avocado that is tender when squeezed, but not soft. You can halve the calories and fat grams per kebab if you omit the avocado. Check the labels when buying mozzarella: most supermarkets now stock reduced-fat varieties, which have approximately half the fat and calories of the full-fat sort.

MAKES 8 KEBABS

Prep: 10 minutes

Per kebab:

100 kcals

418 kJ

6.5g fat

Low GI

8 cherry tomatoes, halved

8 basil leaves

60g/2oz reduced-fat mozzarella, cut into 8 cubes

½ avocado, peeled and stoned (pitted)

a squeeze of lemon juice

sea salt and freshly ground black pepper

1 Thread half a cherry tomato (cut side facing inwards) onto a mini bamboo skewer or wooden cocktail stick (toothpick). Next add a basil leaf and a cube of mozzarella.

2 Cut the avocado into 8 small cubes and squeeze some lemon juice over them to prevent discoloration.

3 Thread one avocado cube onto the skewer followed by another tomato half (cut side facing inwards). Grind a little salt and pepper over the top.

4 Repeat with the remaining ingredients to make 8 kebabs in total. If you're not going to eat them straight away, seal in an airtight plastic container or cover with cling film (plastic wrap) and chill in the fridge for up to a few hours.

TIP: Save the avocado half you are not using by brushing with lemon juice, wrapping in cling film (plastic wrap) and storing for up to 24 hours in the fridge.

PASSIONFRUIT MINI PAVLOVAS

This is the easiest sweet snack or dessert you'll ever make. There's no need to make the meringues yourself – just use the ones you can buy in packs in your local supermarket. If you don't have passion fruit, you can use 150g/5oz fresh raspberries or strawberries instead and the calories will stay the same.

SERVES 2

Prep: 5 minutes

Per serving:

100 kcals

418 kJ

0.1g fat

Low GI

2 passion fruits

3 tbsp 0% fat Greek yoghurt

2 individual meringue nests

1 Cut the passion fruits in half. Scoop out the seeds and juice into a bowl. Discard the hard outer shells.

2 Mix the yoghurt into the passion fruit, swirling it through.

3 Fill the meringue nests with the passion fruit yoghurt and serve.

TIP: You can make these in advance and chill in the fridge for a few hours before eating.

AFFOGATO

Nothing could be quicker and easier to make than this Italian dessert. It's the ultimate flavour experience for real coffee lovers – a fabulous combination of icy cold ice cream and bitter coffee. Ideally, you need a coffee machine or mocha pot that makes really strong espresso – instant coffee doesn't cut it! Check the nutritional information on cartons of 'light' and low-fat ice cream carefully as the calorie content can vary considerably between brands. You're looking for around 60 kcals per 50g/2oz scoop.

SERVES 2

Prep: 5 minutes

Per serving:

100 kcals

418 kJ

3.2g fat

Low GI

120ml/4fl oz (generous ½ cup) strong, freshly made espresso coffee

2 x 50g/2oz scoops low-fat vanilla ice cream

1 square dark (semisweet) chocolate (minimum 70% cocoa solids)

1 Make the coffee in an espresso machine or stove-top coffee maker.

2 Make sure the ice cream is frozen really hard – if it's soft-scoop or semi-frozen it will melt too quickly when you pour the hot coffee over it. Scoop a ball of ice cream into each small bowl or shallow cup.

3 Pour the piping hot espresso coffee over the ice cream and quickly grate the chocolate over the top. Eat immediately before the ice cream melts.

> **TIP:** If you don't have an espresso machine or stove-top pot, make some really strong coffee in a cafetière.

FROZEN YOGHURT STRAWBERRIES

These delicious mini treats are so easy to make and are cooling and refreshing on a warm day. Children love them too and they're much healthier than potato chips, cookies and candy. Other firm fruit from the 'green' list can be used, including blueberries and cherries.

....

SERVES 3

Prep: 10 minutes
Freeze: 2 hours minimum
Cook: 5 minutes

Per serving:

100 kcals
418 kJ
4g fat
Low GI

120g/4oz (generous ½ cup) 0% fat Greek yoghurt

a few drops of vanilla extract

200g/7oz whole strawberries

45g/1½oz dark (semisweet) chocolate chips (minimum 70% cocoa solids)

1 Mix the yoghurt and vanilla extract in a shallow bowl. Holding each strawberry by its stem, lift the leaves up and away from the fruit and dip the tip into the yoghurt. Don't cover the strawberry with yoghurt – you want to show an area of red berry at the top.

2 Carefully arrange the dipped strawberries, leaf-side down and tip-side up, on a wire rack, and place in the freezer. Alternatively, space them out on a baking tray (cookie sheet) lined with baking parchment or waxed paper.

3 Freeze for about 2 hours or until the yoghurt is set and frozen. If there's any yoghurt left over, dip the frozen strawberries again and return to the freezer for another hour.

4 Just before eating, melt the chocolate chips in a heatproof bowl set over a small pan of barely simmering water.

5 Serve the frozen strawberries with the melted chocolate drizzled over the top. The strawberries will keep well in the freezer for a few days and you can eat them as a snack or sweet treat without the chocolate, if wished.

STRAWBERRY *and* LEMON CURD MERINGUE MESS

SERVES 2

Soften: 5 minutes

Prep: 10 minutes

This dessert is a variation on the classic Eton mess but without the cream – perfect for a warm summer's day. Mixed berry or lemon frozen yoghurt also work well, but check the labels and avoid 'creamy' brands. You're looking for a maximum of 100 kcals per 100g/3½oz frozen yoghurt.

Per serving:

190 kcals

795 kJ

1g fat

Low GI

4 x 30g/1oz scoops strawberry frozen yoghurt

6 mini meringues, gently crushed

4 tsp lemon curd

200g/7oz strawberries, sliced (with 2 kept whole for decoration)

2 tbsp 0% fat Greek yoghurt

grated zest of 1 lemon

1 Remove the yoghurt from the freezer about 5 minutes before you start making this, to allow it to soften slightly.

2 Take 2 sundae glasses or dishes and put a scoop of the frozen yoghurt in each one. Sprinkle some of the crushed meringues over the top and drizzle with half the lemon curd.

3 Now add a layer of sliced strawberries. Continue layering up the glasses in this way, finishing with a spoonful of yoghurt and a whole strawberry.

4 Sprinkle with the lemon zest and serve immediately before the frozen yoghurt melts.

FRUIT KEBABS *with* CHOCOLATE SAUCE

A great dessert for chocaholics – the exotic fruit and chocolate sauce combo is irresistible. You can cook these fruity kebabs under the grill (broiler) or loosely wrapped in kitchen foil over hot coals on a barbecue.

SERVES 2

Prep: 15 minutes

Cook: 15 minutes

Per serving:

200 kcals

837 kJ

5.1g fat

Low GI

100g/3½oz ripe papaya, peeled, deseeded and cubed

100g/3½oz fresh pineapple, peeled and cubed

100g/3½oz fresh mango, peeled, stoned (pitted) and cubed

1 small banana, cut into chunks

juice of ½ lemon

1 tsp icing (confectioner's) sugar

For the chocolate sauce:

30g/1oz dark (semisweet) chocolate (minimum 70% cocoa solids)

1 tsp clear honey

2 tsp dark unsweetened cocoa powder

1 tsp cornflour (cornstarch)

120ml/4fl oz (½ cup) water

1 Make the chocolate sauce: put the chocolate, honey and cocoa in a small pan over a low heat until it melts. Meanwhile, in a small bowl, mix the cornflour with a little of the water until smooth. Stir the remaining water into the melted chocolate. Add the cornflour mixture and keep stirring until the sauce thickens and is smooth. Remove from the heat.

2 Preheat the overhead grill (broiler). Thread the pieces of fruit alternately on to 4 wooden skewers (see tip) and place on a foil-lined grill pan. Sprinkle over the lemon juice and dust lightly with the icing sugar.

3 Cook under the hot grill for 5–7 minutes, turning frequently, until the fruit is tender and slightly caramelised. Keep an eye on it to prevent it burning, which will spoil the flavour.

4 Serve the hot kebabs with the warm chocolate sauce.

TIP: Before using the wooden skewers, soak them in water to prevent them burning.

PEACHY CHOCOLATE FILO PARCELS

These crisp little parcels, which only take a few minutes to assemble and cook, are sweet and chocolatey inside. If you eat them with a tablespoon of fat-free Greek yoghurt, add 17 kcals per serving. You can use nectarines or large apricots instead of peaches, and the calories will stay roughly the same.

SERVES 2

Prep: 10 minutes

Cook: 10–15 mins

Per serving:

200 kcals

837 kJ

6.7g fat

High GI

2 x 15g/½oz sheets filo (phyllo) pastry

1 small free-range egg, beaten

2 amaretti biscuits (cookies), crushed

30g/1oz dark (semisweet) chocolate (minimum 70% cocoa solids), grated

1 tbsp 0% fat Greek yoghurt

1 ripe peach, halved, peeled and stoned (pitted)

1 tsp icing (confectioner's) sugar

1 Preheat the oven to 200°C, 400°F, gas mark 6.

2 Lightly brush each sheet of filo pastry with beaten egg. Fold in half by bringing the short edge up and over to meet the opposite short edge. Brush with more beaten egg.

3 In a small bowl, mix together the amaretti, chocolate and yoghurt. Divide between the peach halves, filling the hollow in each.

4 Place a filled peach half in the middle of each filo pastry sheet and bring up the corners to meet at the top in the centre. Pinch the tops together with your fingers to seal them, so they look like a crown.

5 Brush the filo parcels with the remaining beaten egg and place on a baking tray (cookie sheet) lined with baking parchment.

6 Bake in the preheated oven for 10–15 minutes until crisp and golden brown. Serve dusted with icing sugar.

OATY BANANA MUFFINS

These tasty muffins can be eaten at any time of day, even for breakfast when you're in a hurry. They are easy to make and are best served warm.

MAKES 6 MUFFINS

Prep: 15 minutes

Cook: 20–25 minutes

Per muffin:

200 kcals

837 kJ

5.2g fat

Medium GI

50g/2oz (generous ½ cup) porridge (rolled) oats

100g/3½oz (1 cup) plain (all-purpose) flour

1 tsp baking powder

½ tsp bicarbonate of soda (baking soda)

a pinch of ground cinnamon

¼ tsp salt

50g/2oz (¼ cup) light brown sugar

1 large ripe banana (or 2 small ones)

1 large free-range egg, beaten

30g/1oz (2 tbsp) butter, melted

1 Preheat the oven to 180°C, 350°F, gas mark 4. Line a 6-hole muffin tin (pan) with paper cases (muffin cases).

2 Mix together the oats, flour, baking powder, bicarbonate of soda, cinnamon, salt and sugar in a large bowl. Make a hollow in the centre.

3 In another bowl, coarsely mash the banana(s) with a fork and stir in the beaten egg and melted butter.

4 Add the banana mixture to the dry oat mixture and fold through gently with a metal spoon until just combined, without over-mixing. Spoon into the paper cases.

5 Bake in the preheated oven for 20–25 minutes until the muffins are slightly risen and golden brown. You can test whether they are cooked by inserting a skewer into the middle – it should come out clean.

6 Cool a little on a wire rack before serving warm (ideally) or cold. You can store them in an airtight container for 2–3 days.

CHEAT'S TIRAMISU

Tiramisu is usually made with full-fat mascarpone cheese and whipped cream, making it a very high-calorie dessert. However, our cheat's version uses extra light soft cheese and still tastes fantastic at only 200 kcals per serving. Try it and see for yourself.

....

SERVES 2

Prep: 15 minutes

Chill: 1 hour

Per serving:

200 kcals

837 kJ

7g fat

Medium GI

60ml/2fl oz (¼ cup) very hot strong black coffee, e.g. espresso

6 sponge fingers (ladyfingers)

1 free-range egg yolk

1 tbsp caster (superfine) sugar

175g/6oz (¾ cup) extra light soft cheese, e.g. Quark

2–3 drops of vanilla extract

1 tsp dark unsweetened cocoa powder

1 Pour the hot coffee into a bowl and quickly dip 3 sponge fingers into the coffee and divide them between 2 small glass dishes. You must be quick or they will start to fall apart.

2 Beat the egg yolk and sugar with a wooden spoon or electric whisk until really pale, thick and creamy. Beat in the soft cheese and vanilla.

3 Cover the coffee-soaked sponge fingers with half the soft cheese mixture. Now dip the remaining sponge fingers into what's left of the coffee and layer on top of the soft cheese.

4 Cover with the remaining soft cheese, then dust lightly with cocoa powder. Chill in the refrigerator for at least 1 hour to firm up before serving.

CHEAT'S LOW-FAT CARROT CAKE

MAKES 12 SQUARES

Prep: 15 minutes

Cook: 45 minutes

This moist carrot cake is lower in calories and healthier than most commercial ones, many of which are studded with nuts and raisins and covered with cream cheese frosting. You can make a low-fat frosting by mixing 250g/9oz extra light soft cheese with grated orange zest and 2 teaspoons icing (confectioner's) sugar. This will add 30 kcals and 2g fat per serving.

Per square:

200 kcals

837 kJ

11.5g fat

Medium GI

120ml/4fl oz (½ cup) sunflower oil, plus extra for spraying the tin

175g/6oz (scant 1 cup) light brown sugar

3 medium free-range eggs, beaten

225g/8oz carrots, grated

grated zest and juice of 1 orange

175g/6oz (1¾ cups) wholemeal self-raising (self-rising) flour

1 tsp baking powder

1 tsp ground cinnamon

½ tsp grated nutmeg

1 tsp icing (confectioner's) sugar

1 Preheat the oven to 180°C, 350°F, gas mark 4. Lightly spray a 20cm/8in square cake tin (pan) with oil and line with baking parchment.

2 In a food mixer or food processor, beat together the oil, sugar and eggs until well blended. (Alternatively, beat in a large mixing bowl with a hand-held electric whisk.) Mix in the grated carrots and orange zest and juice. Sift in the flour (tipping in any that hasn't gone through), baking powder and spices and stir together thoroughly to mix.

3 Pour the cake mixture into the greased and lined cake tin and smooth the top. Bake in the preheated oven for 45 minutes, or until well risen and a skewer inserted into the centre comes out clean. Leave the cake to cool in the tin.

4 Lightly dust the cold cake with the icing sugar and cut into 12 squares. Store in a covered container in the fridge to keep it moist. It keeps well for 3–4 days.

CHEAT'S BROWNIES

You can enjoy these delicious brownies without having to worry about the calories. Eat as a snack or a dessert, serving each brownie with 60g/2oz fresh raspberries or strawberries and a tablespoon of 0% fat Greek yoghurt. This adds about 40 kcals per serving.

MAKES 9 BROWNIES

Prep: 15 minutes

Cook: 25–30 minutes

Per brownie:

185 kcals

774 kJ

6.5g fat

High GI

125g/4oz (½ cup) reduced-fat sunflower spread, plus extra for greasing

125g/4oz (generous ½ cup) dark molasses or soft brown sugar

2 medium free-range eggs

125g/4oz (1¼ cups) self-raising (self-rising) flour

50g/2oz (½ cup) dark unsweetened cocoa powder

½ tsp baking powder

30g/1oz dark (semisweet) chocolate (minimum 70% cocoa solids), coarsely chopped

125g/4oz (½ cup) virtually fat-free fromage frais

2 tbsp skimmed milk

1 Preheat the oven to 180°C, 350°F, gas mark 4. Grease a 20cm/8in square cake tin (pan) and line the base with baking parchment.

2 Beat the sunflower spread and sugar in a food mixer or with a hand-held electric whisk, until light and fluffy.

3 Beat in the eggs, one at a time, and then sift in the flour, cocoa and baking powder. Beat well then stir in the chocolate and whisk in the fromage frais and milk. You should end up with a smooth cake mixture (batter), which is not too stiff.

4 Pour into the prepared cake tin and level the top. Bake in the preheated oven for 25–30 minutes until cooked and well-risen. Test whether it's cooked by inserting a skewer into the centre – it should come out clean.

5 Leave to cool in the tin and then cut into 9 squares.

CHEAT'S ESPRESSO CHOCOLATE MOUSSE

Our low-calorie chocolate mousse is less than 200 kcals per serving. We've flavoured it with coffee but you could use 2 tbsp freshly squeezed orange juice and some grated orange zest instead – the calories will stay roughly the same. The calorie and fat content of chocolate mousse can vary considerably, with some of the rich versions that you eat in restaurants, made with melted chocolate and thick cream, weighing in at 500 kcals or more per serving.

SERVES 2

Prep: 15 minutes, plus cooling

Chill: 2 hours

Per serving:

180 kcals

753 kJ

8.3g fat

Low GI

---

2 medium free-range eggs, separated

150g/5oz (scant ½ cup) virtually fat-free natural fromage frais

1 tbsp dark unsweetened cocoa powder

2 tbsp very strong, freshly espresso coffee

liquid artificial sweetener, e.g. stevia, to taste

2 tbsp hot water from the kettle

½ sachet powdered gelatine

15g/½oz dark (semisweet) chocolate (minimum 70% cocoa solids)

1 Put the egg yolks and fromage frais in a bowl. Sift in the cocoa powder and stir until smooth. Stir in the espresso coffee and sweeten to taste with artificial sweetener.

2 Pour the hot (not boiling) water into a separate bowl and sprinkle the gelatine over the top. Set aside for 5 minutes, stirring occasionally, until it dissolves. Set aside to cool.

3 Beat the egg whites in a clean, dry bowl until they stand in stiff peaks. Gently fold them into the chocolate mixture in a figure-of-eight movement, using a metal spoon.

4 Stir in the dissolved gelatine, mixing it thoroughly, and spoon into 2 ramekins or glass dishes.

5 Leave to chill in the fridge for at least 2 hours until the mousse is set. Grate the chocolate over the top just before serving.

CHEAT'S APPLE CRUMBLE

Apple crumble is usually made with lots of butter and sugar and averages between 300 and 400 kcals per portion, even more if served with cream or custard. If you don't want to eat our delicious cheat's version plain, you can serve it with 1 tablespoon 0% fat Greek yoghurt and you will add 17 kcals. If you top it with a 60g/2oz scoop of low-fat vanilla ice cream, add 50 kcals and 2g fat.

SERVES 4

Prep: 10 minutes

Cook: 30 minutes

Per serving:

200 kcals

837 kJ

4g fat

Medium GI

400g/14oz cooking (green) apples, peeled, cored and cubed

1 tsp ground cinnamon

a pinch of ground cloves

grated zest and juice of ½ lemon

2–3 tsp granulated sweetener, e.g. stevia

For the crumble topping:

60g/2oz (generous ½ cup) plain (all-purpose) flour

60g/2oz (generous ½ cup) rolled oats (oatmeal)

a pinch of ground cinnamon

30g/1oz (2 tbsp) low-fat spread

2 tbsp Demerara sugar

1 Preheat the oven to 200°C, 400°F, gas mark 6.

2 Put the apples, ground spices, lemon zest and juice in a saucepan and cook gently over a low heat for about 10 minutes, until the apples are just tender but still hold their shape. Sweeten to taste with granulated sweetener.

3 Make the crumble topping: sift the flour into a bowl and stir in the oats and cinnamon. Rub in the low-fat spread with your fingertips until the mixture resembles breadcrumbs. Stir in the sugar.

4 Transfer the apple to an ovenproof dish and cover with the crumble topping. Sprinkle with a few drops of water.

5 Bake in the preheated oven for about 20 minutes, until the top is golden brown and crisp. Serve hot or warm.

TIP: When blackberries are in season, substitute 100g/3½oz of the apples with the same weight in blackberries. Cook the apples as in step 2 and then stir in the blackberries before topping with the crumble.